MW01258207

Purchase this Book Direct At:

www.williamheadapohl.com/SoD/

or

www.createspace.com/3645037

Having snored, snorted, and gasped for air all night
Mr. Apneac drops out of bed, says
"I feel like I've been hit by a Mack truck"
He looks like crap
His wife hates him
His life is a big-fat-bummer
Is that you?


Mrs. Downwind Apneac hasn't slept a wink
She feels psychotic
Again, she dreamt
Of killing him
(In his sleep, just so it will end)
And woke, complaining, rolling over and over,
"H-o-n-e-y, you're snoring!"
Like always, he retorts, "Am not,"
then dodges her elbow,
Though she manages to kick him.
Sleep for her is a big-fat-bummer
Is that you?

## Disclaimer, Caution, & WARNING:

Cover of the book designed by Susan Kare.

Book design and layout by Jon Warren Lentz

Coinage of terms, Apneac, down-wind Apneac, and second-hand snorer, by Jon Warren Lentz

FIRST EDITION

# Sleep or Die

Overcome Apnea Before It Overcomes You

-Three Approaches for Apnea Avengers-

William E. Headapohl

Jon Warren Lentz

# DEDICATIONS

To my dad, sister, and nephew who've all been touched by Apnea. To all my friends with Apnea who are good sports and put up with my constant focus on getting rid of their affliction. And to my eldest sister who, even with busy medical practice, is always up for talking health.

~ W.E.H.


For Rene, who gave me breathing room and whom I love ever true. And for my son, Rob, who inspires me his own sweet brand of devotion and determination.

~J.W.L

# Acknowledgements

Firstly, my huge thanks to Rene Schubert for her tireless research of how the body works, what to eat, what happens with diets, and for running down many theories and ideas critical to the book. I also want to thank my long-time friend and artist Susan Kare for her wonderful cover.

I wish to thank Yoga favorites Kelli Russell and Maura Rassman for being supportive and researching parts of the book as well as Rick Ronald for sharing his surgery stories and not getting his legs cut off. Also my heart-felt thanks to didgeridoo musician and friend Barbara Seymour for exploring the dynamics of Circular Breathing and just hanging out. I also give my kudos to Carol Thompson for inspiring the name for the book name, "Sleep or Die," and for her sage advice, too.

My gratitude to my friend, April Guinchard, for sharing her personal stories and insights as to what a downwind Apneac thinks just might work to motivate another Apneac. Also, author Kurt Starnes for inspiring this book by leading the way with his book; as well as to Gregg Ward, Cynthia Burnham, and Chris Witt for inviting me into their book Mastermind group, even though I was not going to write a book, and then inspiring me to do so. If I wore a hat, I'd take my hat off to printing expert and fellow Positano Rider Tom Andre.

I also want to express my many thanks to industry leader Peter Farrell, founder of ResMed, for being available to me as a sounding board for more than a decade. Also to Mick Farrell for inspiring "predictor zero" in the book–observed cessation of breathing.

I want to express my boundless thanks to my sister, Dr. Dana Headapohl, for all her support and generous reading of the text, and Dr. Lawrence Martin for sharing what makes people change. I also want to give thanks to my other sister, Heidi, for all her sage advice.

It's usually the parents who humor the kids, so I want to give a big nod to my sons, Hunter and Travis Headapohl, who humored me with maturity beyond their years as they ushered me through the writing process as well as for tirelessly giving me their opinions on cover design in between homework. I also want to thank my nephew Levi for inspiring me to realize that I can help others with Apnea.

There may be nothing more difficult than to be the partner of an aspiring writer off to sea on his first book, so let me just share that the gratitude I have for my wife, Carlie, is beyond measure. Thanks!

Finally, but perhaps most of all, as we wrap up this book over Mother's Day weekend, I share my infinite gratitude and respect for my mom, Ruth Headapohl and for going easy on my snoring father who, like me, was touched by Apnea.

~W.E.H. Rancho Santa Fe, CA.

Firstly I want to express my infinite thanks to my fiancé, lover, champion, number one supporter and "bestest" friend, Rene. I want to humbly thank to my co-author, William E. Headapohl, for inviting me to join him on this journey with the ever-clear objective to help others. I would also like to thank all the people listed above who have unknowingly lent me a hand by reaching out to help my friend, Will.

Last but not least I want to acknowledge the infinite power that moved both of us to begin this project and then supported us through more than a year of hard work as Will and I poured countless hours and infinite keystrokes into this project. If this book helps just one person to breathe better and sleep more soundly, it will have been worth it.

~J.W.L. Carlsbad, CA.

# Table of Contents

# INTRODUCTION

## When I Lay Me Down to Sleep...

You shouldn't have to work to go to sleep. You ought to be able to just rest and let sleep come and restore you. But if that's not the case, if sleep does not befriend you, if you are an Apneac, then this book is for you.

### Apnea Avengers

Apnea is best described as evil. Evil with a long-term plan. Apnea slowly and silently insults, ravages, tricks and worsens a body. Experts, who know Apnea, know this; that's why insurance companies refuse individual medical insurance policies to persons with Apnea. They know this particular evil and how it kills their bottom line. Doctors, too, are in the know on this evil. That's why you might hear them pleading, cajoling, browbeating you to take action by losing weight, by exercising "or-else."

That "or-else" is the high probability of a shortened time on earth, of broken relationships, of a lifetime of nights spent face-to-face with a special airflow machine whose only purpose, wheezing through the night, is to keep evil at bay. And sometimes that "or-else" means cutting away at tissue and bone; replacing your face. Medieval evil. Got to keep evil at bay.

Too often, those with this evil creeping up on them are truly the last to know. Denial is evil's cloak. It deceives others as a consequence of their own self-deception. This evil is measured not so much by the magnitude of its sins, but by its relentless persistence.

Yes, Apnea is evil. It must be stopped. It can be stopped.

1

How? How can it be stopped? It starts with a mindset, a simple tenet or belief that you can get better. That you can breathe again. Then you have to decide not to roll over and not to be taken by Apnea, but to fight it with a powerful vengeance like a fury of good.

When you decide to fight it, make the fight so bad-ass-with-good intent, that bad is scared. So powerfully good, that evil leaves to lurk elsewhere - not in your body, and not on your watch. Be asymmetrical in your response; don't just match your opponent blow-for blow, go overboard. You can win. Choose extreme vengeance against Apnea on behalf of your body. But also on behalf of those who share this life with you: your loved ones and family. When you decide to take on this mindset you are thenceforth anointed as another in the growing ranks of Apnea Avengers. Apnea Avengers feel loyalty to their mental and physical health. To let yourself be robbed of life is no longer an option. It's a fight against death and decline. Good and evil. You make good work for you.

Choose wisely: your well-being and your very life depends upon it.

## Snoring and Apnea

This book is about Apnea, a not-so-silent killer. Research shows that if left untreated, Apnea shortens life expectancy by twenty years. If you are over thirty and paying attention, you either know someone who suffers from Apnea or you have it yourself. You or someone you love may have an intuition that something is wrong, but denial is strong like an ox. Too often, the ones with Apnea are the last to know or accept it. Cultures poke fun at snoring, but snoring isn't always a laughing matter; it may be a precursor, a sign that Apnea is lurking around the corner. Not always, but often. **Those with Apnea surely snore but not**

**all snorers have or develop Apnea.** Thus the question; is it Apnea or just obnoxious snoring? This book will help you understand Apnea better.

## Second-Hand Snorers

Eighty-five percent of those touched by Apnea aren't even aware of their disease. These sleep-deprived, undiagnosed sufferers are not getting the treatment that is vitally required to help them avoid a gruesome host of deadly diseases that are known to be spawned by untreated sleep disorder. And for every Apneac, every person who is touched by Apnea, there are many more close friends, relatives, and lovers who are impacted. We call these folks *second-hand snorers* and *downwind Apneacs*. They too are at risk. Why? Because, like everyone else, downwind Apneacs and second-hand snorers also need to sleep or they may develop their own health issues. Even worse, when the untreated Apneac develops an affliction like heart disease or diabetes, or even meets with sudden death, the burden of worry and care falls heavily on the shoulders of family, friends and lovers: the down-wind Apneacs and second-hand snorers.

# A Wake Up Call?

What is Apnea? What are Apnea's menacing variations? Why is Apnea deadly when it's untreated? What makes it such a big-fat-bummer while you are living?

Disturbed sleep and Apnea are bad for everybody. It's a family wrecker and it's a health destroyer. It's also the unrecognized driver behind the wheel of a multitude of afflictions that no one wants to live with. A bump from Apnea can set loose a fleet of chronic sicknesses that are known to shorten lives. Most people are surprised to learn of the incredible punishment Apnea dishes

3

out to all parts of your body. It's not pretty. In the last decade, medical science has slowly and steadily revealed the connections between Apnea and multiple illnesses. For the population at large, it's a bit like the story of cigarettes back in the sixties. Some people require absolute proof, like having every piece of the puzzle in place before they can see the picture. Others can see pattern of the puzzle as it emerges, and they are the lucky ones who step away before they are flattened by the oncoming truck.

# Big-Fat Bummer

Ok, what's a big-fat-bummer? Who isn't familiar with ED (erectile dysfunction) and dual bathtubs on a hillside? Does every guy have it? If you watch US television, it sure seems like they might. Interestingly, with Apneacs it's quite true.

## A Manual for Apnea Avengers

The purpose of this book is to put vital information into the hands of those who want to know more or who need to understand the bigger picture. We want you to get your breath back. The first step is for you to understand that overcoming Apnea is both a process and a continuum. While for some there are simple steps that may help squeeze Apnea away, as if just one piece if the puzzle was required to make a fresh picture. For others it may require a number of steps, because sometimes Apnea is complex puzzle that must be solved entirely before you can back down this dread disease.

Our challenge in writing this book was to help all Apnea-impacted readers with the latest knowledge, tools, and approaches to overcome this killer. In this book we describe various pieces of the puzzle, and we look at many of them from different perspectives, moving step by step through the science and the treatment options, offering you puzzle pieces as you make your way along the continuum. We want to help you to understand the puzzle and to select the tools that will help you or your loved one to overcome Apnea.

## Will's Will

Why do I care? Well, twenty years ago, I traveled around the world. My father agreed to come along for part of the ride. One night along the way, when sleeping in the same room, I was dumfounded, alarmed and confused. I heard my dad as he stopped breathing. I waited, waited and waited until he resumed breathing again. This went on every time we shared a room.

At the time, I had no idea what was going on, and I would never have believed that, on some dark sleep-disturbed night in the future, I would have the same experience. I did not know what Apnea was then, and I had no way of knowing that it was waiting for me, like some evil contagion in my genes.

Then, many years later, after living with Apnea myself for fifteen years, I began to wonder: *I know how to treat Apnea, but why does it happen? If we know why, can we figure out how to overcome it with additional treatments? Might we even reverse Apnea?*

Several years ago, my father passed away from complications related to health afflictions that were likely driven by his Apnea. I'd always wondered why he developed those health afflictions: GERD, heart disease, worsening asthma, then diabetes and, finally, pancreatic cancer. As he was declining, he lost weight, lots of weight. One day, it was one of his final days; he pulled me aside and said, "Hey, I need to tell you something. I don't have Apnea anymore and you need to know this." He'd shed so much weight that now, on his deathbed, he was back again to his high school weight.

And with that, one big piece of the Apnea puzzle was lovingly dropped in my lap. I have my father to thank for this book. Without that heavy-puzzle piece, I might have believed that the puzzle is unsolvable. But it is solvable. Last year, I enlisted my friend Jon to help me put the puzzle into words. This book is our attempt to explain how Apnea can be avenged. ~ W.E.H.

# CHAPTER 1:
# No Sleep Makes You Sick

## *Mack Truck*

*My co-author asked me what it feels like to have Apnea and suggested it might be like a big weight pressing on my chest. I told him that did not sound right. The best I came up with harkens back to a saying when I was a boy. You see, two of my uncles love trucks. They were fond of saying it was "like being hit by a Mack truck." That's the Apnea feeling for me. Since my sleep treatment overcomes my Apnea now, I don't feel that way anymore. Instead, I just drink the cocktail "Mary Got Hit By A Mack Truck." It's easy to make. Combine Diesel brand vodka with Tabasco, tomato juice, pepper, horseradish and salt. It's best to drink while sitting down and then wait for the blow to the head. I'm not really being sarcastic, for Apnea is a far more deadly cocktail than that.*

*~W.E.H.*

## We Are The Travelers

For too many of us a diagnosis of disease is an abstraction. It's just a story, or a myth about a fabled journey having nothing to do with any of us. But then again this story may be tricky; at the end what the tale may really be about is all of the signs that the travelers ignored. The story bumps along with foreshadowing and signs of lurking trouble until finally one sees what spot they've got themselves into, and exclaims, "I am here?" and then, **"Why didn't anyone tell me?"** At the end, we realize we are the travelers. We are the ones who fooled ourselves all along the way. We've ignored the warnings; we have lost the way of health.

## Signs

If you don't read the signs, you won't choose your path wisely; you will be likely to stumble into poor health blindly. Still it's our – or in your case, your – health, and once we realize what's been going on, we can make better choices. Whether you choose to read the rest of this book or not is your choice. Choose wisely. Don't let your disease make the choice for you. You can choose improved health by better understanding your disease. Even if you haven't chosen wisely (donuts over walnuts), or have had bad luck (illness causing nerve damage in the airway), or have bad genes (looks that resemble an Apnea-suffering parent), or are just tired and worn out, **there is hope**. But only you can choose to take control as the owner of your own mind and body. And that means taking responsibility.

## It's All Interconnected

Let's start by talking about trees. It happens that one the world's largest living organisms are a grove of aspen trees. Scientists discovered that the roots of aspen groves are interlinked across miles of mountains, creating a single unified organism sharing the precise same DNA. Killing one edge of the aspen grove is to harm the entire grove. Our human bodies are much like that, except instead of trees we are composed of billions of cells that are all interconnected – and each cell is important to our well-being as a complete organism.

So that means you aren't just a collection of two arms, two legs, some orifices, hair and one or two heads. It all works together and without any one part the entire body suffers and has to rely on an alternative back-up system. Some doctors will tell you that you don't really need this or that organ and probably, sometimes, this is true – especially if the organ is so shot that it's infected or even cancerous. But if it were your organ wouldn't you want to ask more questions?

# Without Breath

Apnea is a serious breathing problem. Also called sleep disturbed breathing, this disease affects not only the Apnea sufferer, or Apneac, but also their families, friends and even colleagues and neighbors. **We call these folks the second-hand snorers, or down-wind Apneacs**: not because it's funny, but because this disease involves others.

## Hope

According to a study published online in the American Journal of Respiratory and Critical Care Medicine, researchers have found that, with early detection, followed by treatment with CPAP (continuous positive airway pressure), the brain changes caused by OSA are at least partially reversible. So if you think you or your partner may have Apnea, get help sooner than later in order to avoid or possibly reverse the worst.

As for the Apneacs themselves, untreated, Apnea can rob them of restorative sleep and make them very sick. No sleep as a result of no breathing can be the driver of additional chronic diseases, including top killer diseases like diabetes and cardiovascular disease.

# Sleep or Die

That's right, "Sleep or Die." We titled this book to address the bottom-line; eventually, Apnea calls all of its victims to account. Just talk to widows and widowers. We have. A family friend who had recently lost her husband to heart disease driven by OSA, just netted it out one day when asked what to call this book. After being presented with a set of lovely names that invoked the "beauty of breathing well and the heightened awareness and engagement in life, " She blurted out "Sleep or Die. Don't beat around the bush."

## CPAP Era

While people have suffered from Apnea for centuries, Apnea generally went untreated and so led to or compounded other health problems, which often led to an early death. Even the tracheotomy, which was one method of intervention in extreme Apnea, had the frequent complication of death from infection. It wasn't until the early 80's that Dr. George Gregory and colleagues in the neonatal intensive care unit at the University of California, San Francisco developed a CPAP (continuous positive airway pressure) pump and breathing mask. Then a variation of the CPAP system was developed by Professor Colin Sullivan at Royal Prince Alfred Hospital in Sydney, Australia. The era of hope began.

## Apnea Defined

The word Apnea (or *apnoea* in some journals) is Greek and means, literally, without breath. A clinical diagnosis of Apnea is rendered when a patient's breathing stops completely five or more times each hour, during "sleep." Diagnosed or not, this fact cannot be overemphasized: **untreated Apnea has long-term debilitating consequences and leads to other diseases**. Hypopnea is a related state that occurs during "sleep" when breathing has not totally stopped but is reduced to a point where little air is flowing; then the normally oxygen-rich blood becomes more and more depleted until it reaches dangerously low levels.

Both Apnea and Hypopnea result from one or more obstructions of the airway, which runs from the tip of the nose to the lungs. These two cousins, Apnea and Hypopnea, both impact the body in a very negative way, inflicting increasing damage over time.

## Measuring Apnea

The measurement most often used to diagnose sleep disturbed breathing is the Apnea-Hypopnea index, which is commonly abbreviated as the AHI.

It is also the key measurement used by doctors and others, such as employers in industries where wakefulness is imperative (like trucking), to describe the severity of the disease.

## A Deadly Cocktail

Apnea has been aptly described as a deadly cocktail that mixes your inheritance and your choices; that's **one-part inherited traits and one-part lifestyle choices**. The inherited traits involve the anatomy of the upper airway, particularly what's readily visible in the neck and face, while the lifestyle part

11

involves self-inflicted burdens developed from diet, exercise and occupation as well as other choices we make in our lives, such as drinking, smoking, or the number of hours spent glued to the television.

## Your Control

As the authors of this book it's our job to point out that a number of the factors that can lead to a healing of Apnea are, in fact, within the control of any Apneac; they are already in your TOOLbox. Factors such as muscle tension, tone, sleeping position, degree of obesity, substance use, are all well within the control of any Apneac. Sure, it may not be dead easy to take control, but then is your own death a better outcome? We intend to show you how to take control and to support you in your own progress towards handling and healing your disease.

Inherited traits predispose a person to Apnea by creating an environment where lifestyle choices can determine whether those traits lead to full-blown Apnea. For example, a person may have an inherited trait whereby their tongue is a bit too big for their mouth or perhaps an airway that is unusually small. Usually, this won't be a problem. But such traits, when combined with lifestyle choices that lead to excessive fatty tissue surrounding the neck, can throw the Apnea switch, developing into sleep-deprived breathing initially begun by relatively mild symptoms of reduced oxygen during sleep. This is the beginning that leads to a vicious cycle of life-threatening proportions.

## The Run Down

Apnea is serious. But if you had Apnea, would you know it? According to the statistics, it's not likely that you would know. In fact, **over 85% of Apnea sufferers don't even know they have it!** Too often, all they know is that they are tired and they feel like they have been "run over by a truck." These sufferers are quite likely to know the names of all of the other chronic diseases they may have; like heart disease, ADHD or diabetes, but most of them will be shocked to learn that their "poor sleep" results from the cessation of breathing. Nearly all of them will be dumfounded when they learn that **a person with Apnea can stop breathing thirty times an hour**, all night long, and still not know they have it. Consequently, most Apneacs are entirely unaware that their other deadly chronic diseases – such as heart disease or diabetes type II – are due to oxygen deprivation caused by the poor sleep that Apnea renders.

## There is Hope

We now interrupt this ceaseless lament to tell you that there is hope. That is, after all, why we wrote this book. **Medical studies have shown success with a number of approaches**. There are viable nonsurgical approaches, device therapies like CPAP, some noninvasive to minimally invasive treatments, and of course, surgeries. Taken together we call this, "The Apnea Avenger's TOOLbox"

## There is No Silver Bullet

We've organized three approaches to the overarching theme of this book, which is that you can and should "overcome Apnea before it overcomes you." But how? That's the question, the question that's literally taken our breath away. There is no magic answer. For most, it's quite likely that past efforts to become healthier have not been met with lasting success.

One-off efforts to get a handle on a chronic condition like Apnea too often fall short. But this time it may be different. We've found that it's the nature of Apnea, for which there is no single solution, no silver bullet, that it requires a coordinated and thoughtful approach. This is where selecting the right TOOLs for the job comes into play. When you decide to go from Apneac to Apnea Avenger, you'll get there with these TOOLs.

# TOOLs

To make our TOOLs approach easier for Apnea Avengers to understand, we're going to describe three approaches as though they are drawers in a TOOLbox. Just as a professional mechanic organizes TOOLs in a logical way, sorting and storing them according to purpose or theme – as, for example, a drawer for screwdrivers, another for wrenches, for hammers, drills, and so on: whatever the approach to organization, a well-organized TOOLbox is a logical place to keep the TOOLs so that they are there when you need them.

And that is exactly what we've done with the Apnea Avenger's TOOLs. We've organized the TOOLs by purpose or theme into three TOOLbox drawers. This way the Apnea Avenger, armed with knowledge, will be empowered to select the right TOOLs to get the job done. A complete rebuild may involve the selection and implementation of multiple TOOLs, while a simple fix might need just one. It depends as much on the individual breathing issue itself as on the desired outcome. So, before we get started, let's take a look at our Apnea Avenger TOOLbox. It has three drawers with two or more TOOLs in each drawer.

✓ **External TOOLs** drawer– With this approach, Apnea Avengers use external TOOLs (someone or something else) that are not naturally part of the body. They are either worn, strapped on, or are modifications made to the body. External TOOLs work on either the entire system or on specific systems or parts of the body. Surgery and CPAP are examples of the TOOLs found in the External TOOLs drawer.

✓ **System TOOLs** drawer – With this approach, Apnea Avengers rely upon themselves to use TOOLs of knowledge and motivation to make changes to the entire bodily system. Weight Loss and Global Exercise are examples of the TOOLs found in the System TOOLs drawer.

✓ **Targeted TOOLs** drawer– With this approach, Apnea Avengers rely upon TOOLs that empower them to take targeted actions, including specialized exercises, to drive specific outcomes intended to change specific parts of the body. Circular Breathing, playing a musical instrument such as the Didgeridoo, Oropharyngeal Exercises, Isometric Gum-chewing, and Targeted Yoga are all examples of the TOOLs found in the Targeted TOOLs drawer.

Now before we can get into these approaches to treating and perhaps even healing Apnea, we're going to invest substantial time – and ink – several chapters in fact, to describe what Apnea is all about, how bad it can get, and what horrible outcomes are often associated with it. **Knowledge is power, but information without solutions can also be frustrating.** We intend to appease your frustrations with both knowledge and solutions.

15

So, before we delve into the approaches we've organized in the Apnea Avenger's TOOLbox, we're going to give you the information and knowledge you'll want (and need) in order to make best use of the TOOLs in this book. But we'll also do our best to make this an easy and entertaining read. Not quite Three Stooges hilarity, nuk-nuk, but don't be surprised if we drag a belly laugh out of you from time to time.

## Neck, Neck

There is more good news. Our Apnea research has identified a surprising common denominator: **the severity of a person's Apnea is correlated to their neck size.** This is a key finding: With neck-targeted-exercise or diet, resulting in reduced neck circumference, the severity of Apnea was also reduced. Thus, as neck circumference is now understood to be a primary driver of Apnea, the reduction of neck circumference is recognized to play a primary role in reversing Apnea. Simply stated, this means that Apnea sufferers who are willing to make the effort can expect a lessening of their symptoms and an easing of their condition; in the best circumstances this may even lead to a reversal of Apnea.

The significance of neck circumference, and the studies that underlie these claims, will be discussed in greater detail throughout the rest of this book.

## Do I Just Snore, Or Do I Have Apnea?

Now there are a couple of crucial questions that must be addressed. You are wondering, **do I just snore or do I have Apnea?** Here's the other question, **does your partner's snoring really add up to Apnea or are you too easily bothered?**

The answer to the first question will be found in the chapters of this book. The second question is a little easier to answer, but no less involved: usually it is your partner's Apnea– you are not crazy. But then, you just might go crazy. News stories tell of partners blaming their Apneac sleeping partner for losing control and the late night domestic havoc that resulted.

Experience and extensive research bear out the brutal fact that Apnea is not an individual problem. These are another class of suffers: second-hand snorers and down-wind Apneacs. Over time, snoring and Apnea can become an enormous aggravation and source of discord. In too many cases, **Apnea is a family wrecker**. Why should that be your future?

## Does Apnea Halve YOU?

Do you take ownership of Apnea? Do you have it? Or does it have you, and is it killing you by halves? No matter how you spin it, identification is key. Here are symptoms to watch out for:

- ✓ Even after eight hours of sleep, you don't feel rested.

- ✓ As the day wears on, you feel more and more tired; by afternoon you want a nap.

- ✓ You know that your loud, habitual snoring disturbs others.

- ✓ Your bed partner reports stops in your breathing.

- ✓ In any of these scenarios, you wake-up feeling half rested, half alive, as though a truck had run over you again and again, halving your night between gasping and sleeping.

## Oxygen

As you will learn in this book, OSA and the resulting lack of oxygen in your body wreaks havoc on multiple organs. Equally, lack of oxygen is impacting organs critical to life and to quality of life; a properly functioning heart is obviously critical but a responsive erection goes a long way, too... Oh yes, as you will see, OSA touches even the least obvious parts of the body. We can take lots of punches; we cannot maintain ourselves for very long without rich oxygenated blood.

# Respiration De-Mystified

Breath is not optional. So when it comes to breathing troubles, it is helpful to understand the pieces of the puzzle. By definition, Obstructive Sleep Apnea means you are not going to have enough oxygen in your blood for a substantial part of each night. This is called oxygen saturation and it is measured as a percentage. When the oxygen saturation level dips below normal levels of between 96% and 99%, stress on the body tissues increases. With Apnea event, the saturation level can dip dangerously low – often below 90%.

Human respiration occurs in four stages:

✓ Moving the air in and out of the alveoli of the lungs. The alveoli are tiny tree-like structures in the lungs. This is called ventilation.

✓ Exchange of gases between the alveoli and the capillaries in the lungs. This is referred to as pulmonary gas exchange.

18

&#10003; The movement of the gases through the circulation of blood to the outer capillaries in organs. This is called gas transport.

&#10003; The exchange of gases in the tissues. Here, carbon dioxide gas is taken away and the cells accept the oxygen. This is termed peripheral gas exchange.

During an Apnea event, air is not allowed to come in or out of the lungs and the respiration cycle is disrupted. This is called hypoxia, meaning that the body tissues are deprived of an adequate oxygen supply. Adequate oxygen supply is most critical to the brain. Continuous episodes of disrupting the oxygen supply can create damaging effects throughout the body.

OSA is insidious. Sneaky. It causes our bodies to sense, *something is very wrong*, alerts us to wake and breathe, and then allows us to retreat back to sleep and repeat the cycle all night long. **Visualize an evil person covering your mouth with a pillow twenty times an hour.** Not quite long enough for us to die, but long enough for us to kick in our emergency wake-up system. Some equate this to torture. Evil? Yes. It's aimed at you. Clever? Yes, because you can't recall it happening. Dangerous? Absolutely. One misfire in your emergency wake-up system spells death. Visualize hanging on by a thread. Some folks have a strong thread and can muscle though a lifetime of the insults; others are not as strong and succumb to an event that can forever change their well-being or their survival on earth.

## Overcome Apnea: It's a Mindset

We get to unhealthy by ignoring signs and generally not taking care of our health. How do we know this? We are human. Like nearly all of us, we have to learn the hard way about taking better care of our own health.

## Make it Personal

This is my problem; I am responsible for fixing it. That's a mindset worth having. Why? Because your doctor owns your problem only partially, usually for about fifteen minutes while face to face with you in their office. Consider this: if a doctor sees twenty patients a day or four hundred in a month, then how special are you?

Don't misunderstand. Doctors care, but they aren't with you 24 hours a day. With Apnea, you retain your sleep problem eight hours every night, and you live the adverse health consequences throughout your life.

Successfully overcoming an affliction takes a certain way of thinking, a mindset of "I own my problem." Then you hold it and solve it, gleaning knowledge from many sources, including this book. Use this information to become an educated and empowered patient, and then actively partner with your doctor to avenge this deadly disease.

### Fix Me! Fix Me! I Am Over Here ... Fix Me!

Historically, the western medical system has perpetuated an atmosphere where patients hand over the key to their health. It's so easy. Usually, it's a magic pill. And, in so many cases they really are like magic. We seek medical attention only after we've run off the rails of good health.

The dialog goes like this; "Wow, I missed the signs and did not see this coming. What can you prescribe for me?" Unfortunately there is no pill yet for Apnea.

A fundamental shift is in the health care system is in the works. The US medical "supply chain" is breaking. Costs are going up while the doctors' portion of the fee is going down. Although still a critical part of the system, doctors have a difficult future. Doctors are in "the squeeze." You will be, too, as more doctors abandon private practice and strike employment deals with hospital organizations. That's because the big medical systems have rules of engagement. Like the legal profession, doctors' hours have to be billable. **When a doctor devotes time to coaching an Apneac to reverse OSA, it's not a billable event.** And that's why you are on your own. It's also why surgery and medical devices are prescribed by the medical world. They are billable.

Luckily, many of those devices, like CPAP, work well at *controlling* OSA. But if you want to reverse or eliminate OSA, CPAP is not the right tool. Some surgeries may work sometimes; at best they can reverse Apnea, but often surgery fails to significantly reduce Apnea, or does so just temporarily. Great minds everywhere are focused on getting our medical health care system right. But in the meantime, your "great mind" needs to take care of Numero Uno.

## You Are Numero Uno

Get your head-neck-and-heart around this: "These are MY cells and it's my job to protect them." Everybody has a boss. You are the boss of your cells and your life force. They all want to do the right thing. You need to lead them. Ever had a group of employees give up on you? It happens. Cells can give up on your too. Don't let them. Take charge!

Making changes in life is simple... it's just not easy. By the end of this book, hopefully you will see how overcoming Apnea can be simple. The prescription is not that complicated, as you will see. So here's that first step, getting started: Nudge yourself. Simply begin with a few small immediate changes, and change becomes easy. **Healthy change gains momentum.** Don't we all find that to be true? And healthy habits, especially exercise and wholesome meals in appropriate portions, support you to feel better. That, in turn, enables you to exercise more, thereby generating an appetite for more healthy foods, and all that in turn leads to health and betterment.

When you take such action, and you change pivotal habits, your body benefits; then you feel happier in your healthy habits and the change is reinforced. You can notice it yourself. **This book will help you identify TOOLs that you can use, change or adjust.** For example, how you exercise and the quality and quantity of your meals are both TOOLs, which are already within reach, and which could-would-should be used in an active (not passive) approach to the treatment and healing Apnea.

Even surgery, which is normally considered a passive approach, can become an active choice, when chosen as the proper resort in a context of knowledgeable exhaustion of other alternatives.

Using and adjusting the simple TOOLs that match your circumstances, you can change your feelings (most Apneacs experience a degree of hopelessness about their disease – hence, the denial) and begin to heal of your own body.

From there, it's a virtuous cycle that improves the quality of your life. It can become easy work, a well-worn path – but it takes a determined mindset.

Read on!

# CHAPTER 2:
# Breathless Geeks

## *On the Brink of Violence*

*Living in San Francisco during the dotcom era, my wife
and I banded together with about five families to rent a
ski cabin each season. Every year, the mix shifted as
some families dropped out and new families popped in.
In the late 90's a new couple joined. The schedule was
a little chaotic which led to occasional overlaps. Having
not begun to use a CPAP nor had my Apnea-related-
tongue surgery yet, plus carrying extra pounds, I was a
loud snorer; freight train quality.*

*One memorable weekend, all the rooms were taken
and the "new guy," was told he'd be bunking in the
same room with me, since our families had stayed
home. He was not happy, at all. I warned him that I
snored, but I was in denial about how loud. After a night
of loud yelling and tossing things my way, the new guy
stormed out. Next morning, it nearly came to blows. A
decade later the new guy is still mad.*

*~W.E.H.*

# Apnea Basics

It's unavoidable. Someone who sleeps with a facemask and pump, dressed like an astronaut is likely to look like a geek. But it's not just about embarrassment or vanity. It's serious.

If you just picked this up and began reading it, likely either you or someone you know snores or are short of breath. You want answers because inspiration is required. **This is a health problem that has seemed insurmountable. Until now**. In the previous chapter, we began to introduce the issues surrounding Apnea, and began to explain that there is hope for Apneacs. Beyond treatment by surgery or the abatement of symptoms through a lifetime of bedtimes dressed like an astronaut in a CPAP mask, there are other things you can do to reduce your suffering, or even heal. In this chapter we begin to break down the causes of Apnea and begin to introduce the concept of options, because there are TOOLs that you can use.

## Untreated and Dead

Untreated Apnea is associated with increased risk of high blood pressure, heart attack, irregular heartbeat, heart failure, and stroke – plus death from any of these causes or in combination with these causes. Treated or untreated, Apnea is linked with obesity and diabetes. It's also linked to excessive daytime sleepiness, which increases the risk of injuries and death from drowsy driving and other accidents, while also lowering performance in the bed, the workplace and at school. Untreated, Apnea is a bummer and a killer.

# Three Kinds of Apnea

**When a person wakes five or more times per hour with OSA events, they are clinically diagnosed with Apnea.** There are three basic forms of Apnea: Obstructive Sleep Apnea, Central Sleep Apnea and Mixed Sleep Apnea, which may also be referred to as CompSA. The general, non-specific term, Apnea, is generally used to cover all three.

## Obstructive Sleep Apnea

The first and most common form of Apnea is Obstructive Sleep Apnea (OSA). It's named obstructive because with this form of Apnea, the stoppage of breath occurs when a sleeper's airway collapses or is blocked by the tongue. Roughly 84% of all Apnea sufferers are diagnosed with this form of Apnea - OSA.

## Central Sleep Apnea

Central Sleep Apnea (CSA) without OSA affects just under 1% of the total Apnea population. Yet the statistical insignificance belies the extreme dangers of this form of the disease. With CSA, the brain forgets to tell the body to breathe. Healthy sleepers rely on correct sensing of both oxygen and C02 and on complicated brain signals to control breathing. CSA represents a disastrous malfunction.

## Mixed Sleep Apnea

While around 84% of Apneacs have OSA, and another 1% have CSA, what do we call the form of Apnea that stalks the other 14%? It's Mixed Events or Mixed Apnea. Just as it sounds, the Mixed Apnea sufferer has a combination of OSA and CSA

## Terminological Confusion

Although Obstructive Sleep Apnea is often referred to as OSA, in the literature it's often shortened to Apnea. Central Sleep Apnea is spelled out completely or else shortened to CSA. We find that Mixed Sleep Apnea is referred to as Mixed, Mixed Apnea, or Mixed Events; yet the acronym MSA is not in common use. According to context, Apnea may refer to all three variants of sleep disturbed breathing, or just OSA. In this book, we attempted to abide by the observed inconsistent conventions of the Apnea literature, with occasional redundancies to make things clear.

# A World of Apnea Sufferers

We have no way to estimate, much less calculate, the number of Apnea sufferers in the world. Nor are there sufficient statistics to begin to compare the incidence of Apnea in the industrialized world to other societies. According to the National Institute Health we know that, **in the US alone, there are at least 20 million OSA sufferers**. According to Resmed Inc., a premier supplier of CPAP machines worldwide, the US number with sleep disordered breathing tops 40 million (including all variations of Apnea). Whether it's 20 or 40 million, we find that only 20% are diagnosed. So in the total US population of 312 million, between 6% and 12% (that's 52-104 million people) suffer with a form of Apnea, while only a fifth of them are getting a diagnosis, much less help. That's a lot of suffering.

## James?

We Asked, "CPAP... Would James Bond Wear One?"
Here are the answers:

- ✓ If he wanted to look cool, at a SEAL Team dress-up party, it's a toss-up between CPAP and a Jet pack.

- ✓ If Bond waited long enough and felt crappy enough, tried a CPAP provided by "Q" and then felt unbelievably ever more super spy, then yes.

- ✓ If he still wanted "Ms. Galore," and if she told him to, then yes of course, he would – but secretly.

- ✓ If 007 were into denial, he would hide his Apnea, always leaving the woman before sneaking off-screen to snort in his sleep, alone.

How can we understand the extent of this epidemic? Sometimes it's helpful to look around. A typical Southwest Air Boeing 737-300 has around 130 passengers in second-class. This means 8 to 16 flyers on every plane are likely to have Apnea. With 23 rows and using the high number of 16, there's one Apneac in every-other-row. Of these 16 Apneacs, only three are diagnosed and or getting treatment, while the other 13 blissfully ride along, tiredly trending toward early chronic illness.

# Second-hand Snorers and Down-wind Apneacs

For just about every Apneac, there is a spouse, partner or lover impacted by Apnea. (Even roommates count.) Second-hand snorers and down-wind Apneacs are included in the suffering because either their own sleep is directly curtailed, or perhaps they find themselves tasked to care for the Apneac. Using conservative figures, **simple math puts 40 to 80 million Americans in the down-wind Apneac impact zone**. It doesn't have to be that way. There is hope. There are TOOLs to help.

## Partner's Lament

At 1:30 am, I sit in bed listening to my husband sleep. It goes something like this: normal sleeping and occasional snoring, the snoring gradually gets louder. He stops breathing for what seems like forever although it is only seconds. Then he starts again. This when I begin listening and noticing. Then he snores loud and then louder and even louder than before, then no breathing at all. After a few seconds, he stumbles to find breath, again. Not only is this a nuisance, since it's keeping me up, it is terrifying; my darling husband, the father of my baby, is not breathing well.

**"To inspire" is to breathe in. To be inspired in response to a diagnosis of Apnea is to inhale hope and to seek a path that will lead you or your loved one away from illness and towards health.**

# Approaches for Overcoming Apnea

In later chapters we develop three groups, or drawers of TOOLs that can be useful to Apnea. But for now, just so you'll understand what we mean by TOOLs, here's a story: Imagine you are moving down the path of life cruising along, steering the wheel of this vehicle called, "your health." For now, let's just imagine this vehicle runs on sunlight and has one large TOOL or control – the steering wheel – and that when you turn the wheel to the left or to the right you are steering into twin ditches of sickness and ill health. But if, quite literally on the other hand, you choose differently and steer down the middle, mindfully staying on the highway of good health, then you are moving along to health and fitness because of your constant attention to choices. The steering wheel can be considered a TOOL that can be adjusted either separately or in synergy with other TOOLs, like a navigational system, or a two-way radio, in order to help you make your best effort to stay on the road and, over time, to heal.

## It's Not You Alone

Apnea is not an individual problem. You aren't driving solo. In most cases Apnea is a family wrecker. Why should that be?

As the travelers, we have heard about the signs on the road that warn us about what is ahead. Use the TOOLS. Read the danger ahead and respond to the changing byway. Paying attention to the signs and steering is critical, because ignoring them will allow the heavyweight, Apnea, to smash the breath right out of you.

We've heard Apneacs say that, for them, sleeping is like getting run over by a truck. **"When you wake-up in the morning, you don't know that you weren't breathing; all you know is that it feels like a Mack truck has run you over. On a bad morning, you'd swear that the truck backed up over you, just for good measure."** Apnea is so evil that it masks the very reality of its intrusion in your life. You don't know that you weren't breathing. You do not understand how dangerous your nights have become.

The alternative is for travellers to respond to the warning signs, and just as staying in your lane helps to ensure that a truck won't run you over, you can use the TOOLs we provide in this book to either protect or restore your health. Signs are critical. With Apnea the signs can sometimes be blurry or faint. Other times, they are right in your face. It depends. But there will be signs. We hope reading this book will give you an increased ability to see and read the signs, and to help you to know how to respond and what TOOL to use.

## Breath of Life: Spiritual, Inspire, Inspiration

Yoga, meditation, martial arts and many other practices focus on the breath in order to access higher levels of the discipline. That's because breath affects us on a cellular level and across all dimensions of our being. You can have ready evidence for yourself. Do an experiment, right now. Take a deep breath. Let it out. Do it again. Notice now, as you take two or three really deep breaths, the breathing changes you. Your awareness may change. Or there may be changes in the feeling of your body. As you open to it, your breath may even help you to be more appreciative. It's a continual miracle that affects us, sustains us, on a cellular level. It is a reminder to every part of you, of the gift of life that is happening in you right now.

# Every Apneac Snores, But Not All Snorers Have Apnea

What we hear is a lot of snoring, snorting, and gasping. Data from the Wisconsin Sleep Cohort Study found that 44 percent of all men surveyed and 28 percent of all women surveyed were habitual snorers. Overall, only 4 percent of the men and 2 percent of the women had snoring that was associated with Apnea. Lots of people snore.

## The Snoring End of The Funnel

If you are alert to developments in the health and medical stats, you're likely to be alert to the fact that the incidence of Apnea is at an all-time high; not just in terms of numbers, but in growing proportion to the total population. We see it as a progression or continuum, as the obvious outcome of an epidemic of snoring. Think of a funnel. At the snoring end of the funnel there are literally millions upon millions merely losing sleep as their health worsens and they gradually progress towards undiagnosed Apnea, bringing them closer and closer to the clinical definition of the disease. Until, finally, they arrive at the narrow end of the funnel where millions of Apneacs suffer the ravages of ruined sleep, slowly succumbing to the correlated afflictions that accompany it.

The good news for habitual-snorers and heavy-snorers is that the TOOLs offered in this book can knock down snoring. Plus it's easier to reverse snoring than reverse full-blown OSA. It's akin to skiing steep moguls and then moving down to the intermediate slopes. It's much easier having mastered advanced techniques on the steep stuff. Slight to moderate snoring are the blue slopes but OSA reversal requires mastery of the TOOLs and skills to ski the black diamonds. As every skier knows, lots of people can do black diamonds. It just takes the right TOOLs and the right mindset.

## What is Habitual Snoring?

Heavy snoring? Or Apnea. So what's going on? Heavy snoring is both a symptom and a predictor of Apnea itself. **If you snore, you may eventually develop Apnea. If you have Apnea, you already snore.**

# Breathless Greek

Remember, the word "Apnea" is a Greek word. Actually a very precise combination of two words, it means "without breath." This will be on the test. Is your life just a test? Or is this the real thing? A life without breath?

Often the sufferer's partner will report that, "He wakes up in the night gasping." Or that, "I never sleep anymore ... but then neither does he." Whereupon her husband will joke, as he perhaps makes pig noises, saying, "Yup, my own snorting keeps me awake." Conversations like this are symptoms of two things: the first is Apnea, denial is the second. **The problem with this health-related denial is that it's like driving while ignoring many important signs along the road of health.** The problem with denial of Apnea is that it's a killer and like driving half asleep; it's also a high stakes game: not just for you but your whole family. Your whole family is at risk. Even if there never is an accident, which is a statistical improbability, or an operation, or a job loss, Apnea is still a family wrecker.

## Read On

As you continue reading, we are going to tell you what's going on with Apnea and then we're going to teach you to use your brain to tell your muscles how to obtain tone in order to deal with your Apnea so that you can begin to heal yourself. As you read, we ask that you listen to your heart. Not just the physiological heart in your chest upon which your life depends, but also the heart that knows how many others depend on you for the quality of their lives. Read on for you own life, but also for those who share in your life.

## The Mind/Heart Connection

A good friend of Will's, an acupuncturist and breath therapist, is fond of saying, "Your head and your heart are vying for control, and the neck is the battle ground." Think of Apnea as a manifestation of this. The neck is the structure upon which the mind resides and rides; the neck is the conduit for signals, nourishment, and the oxygen that fires our thoughts. It's critical for a balanced body.

Perhaps Apnea is more than just a sign that the neck is in trouble. We know that Apnea is rough on our hearts. **Could it be the heart's way of saying, stop the flawed thinking that leads to eating poorly, smoking heavily, and not exercising?** As long as our linear western mindset rejects such a ridiculous notion, we will never know ... or maybe we already know, and what we know is Apnea?

## A Muscle to Move Forward

Exercising muscles makes them smarter, quicker and toned. Exercising a muscle also strengthens the muscle's connection with the brain and fosters better and more-robust neural connections. So we invite you to exercise your brain and consider how a muscle can lift the weight of Apnea off your chest. **Consider which muscle really lifts that spoon of ice cream to your mouth. Is it not your brain?** Remember, you are in control.

# If I Should Die Before I Wake . . .

Over a period of four to five years, the nighttime breathing disorder known as Apnea increases a person's risk of having a heart attack or dying by 30%. Research also shows that people with Apnea who died suddenly from arrhythmia tended to die more during sleep, unlike other heart disease patients whose sudden deaths tend to happen in the few hours after waking up.

Doctors tell Apneacs not to take sleep aids or other medications that can prevent waking up. That's because the emergency wake-up system can fail under that influence, and trouble can ensue. You might wake-up dead.

Much of this book, "Sleep or Die," is nourishment for your brain, a series of explanations for your mind, brain TOOLs, so that it can train all of your other muscles; and specifically train the muscles that are involved in Apnea. The muscles that you need to exercise to ease and relieve Apnea are the muscles that want to hear from your brain; they want to hear, "I am closely aware of your needs and connected. I will choose not to deprive you of oxygen."

Advanced science supports the notion that Apnea may partially result from an impaired connection between the brain and the neck muscles, and that they need a stronger connection to the brain in order to not collapse when sleeping. Although further direct medical research is needed in this area, advances in our understanding of neuroplasticity and exercise physiology support the concept. **Specific exercise may rewire lost connections to neurons and also recruit other neurons as alternate pathways that can be used to replace damaged ones.** Studies with mice show that damaged neurons in the brain allowed airway collapse to occur at night while asleep. Apnea was quick to occur, resulting in a further spiral of decline related to OSA, until eventual death.

The growing science of neuroplasticity shows that this kind of damage can be rewired in much the same way that a modern stroke victim is helped to relearn how to use a limb.

When co-author Jon's right arm was nearly severed and re-attached, he focused his mind to coax new neural pathways across knotted scar tissue and regain the use of a hand that surgeons had told him would be forever useless. In fact, he just typed those lines with both hands.

## Don't Take Your Brain for Granted

While on earth, mental capacity and acuity make a difference in our experience of a full life. Until taken away, it's easy to take your mental gifts for granted. Yet sudden changes are easy to note, as in the case of a concussion. You'll never hear a football player say "I prefer to feel groggy and in a fog. That headshot was the best."

With OSA, the brain injury gathers slowly but with similar results: feeling in a fog, like a truck hit you, depressed, confused and cognitively compromised. **Medical studies have shown conclusively that OSA can, and often does, lead to a reduction of grey matter in the brain – and that is the part that thinks!** No one is likely to agree that would be preferable. So before this happens to you, change course, listen with your entire being and value a clear functioning consciousness; choose to heal. Get ahold of some TOOLs.

## Don't Take Your Breathing for Granted

Breathing and sleep have a common thread. No one thinks much about either of one. We just assume they will continue without need for maintenance. Luckily, for the most part, they do. But as we all know, everything has a limit. Push your body past its adaptive nature and dysfunction results. Our western approach to sleep is to just "fit it in." But we are learning, especially those of us with Apnea, that sleep really is "a main event." **We are learning about what is now called, in the sleep circles, "Good sleep hygiene."** We are learning that sleep is crucially important to how we feel and function during that other main event called, "the waking hours." You can maintain your life. Overcoming OSA is mostly a maintenance issue. Otherwise, if ignored and left to progress with its evil plan, OSA certain to spawn ugly offspring in the form of one of many dread diseases far worse than simply feeling like you've been hit by a truck every morning.

Get healthy sleep. Breathe in, breathe out, and repeat.

No more of this "pausing of breathing" nonsense.

Your body can't tolerate it and you don't have to either.

Choose for yourself. Read on!

# CHAPTER 3:
# Steer Clear

## *How Bad it Can Get*

*In my first career I worked as a sculptor pioneering sand-carved glass as a medium for abstract fine art. In 1989 I fell with a piece of my work as I was leaving an art gallery in San Francisco. Sliding across the top of my right arm, a twenty-pound glass shard severed muscles, nerves and tendons to the bone. I remember waking sedated in a hospital bed, surrounded by doctors. I was a teaching event. One doctor held up my arm pointing and tugging at the bandages. "This guy did the worst thing possible to his arm. Everything across the back of his forearm was severed. As we know, nerves do not grow back. He will never regain the full use of his hand because those are the critical connections for grip and dexterity." Enraged, I grabbed the doctor's arm with my left hand, saying, "Thank you, doctor, for your help. But don't plaster me with your limitations. You did your part. The rest will be up to me. I'll come back some day to prove you wrong."*

*Things worsened. Following the Santa Cruz earthquake, I lost my studio, home, and family. I truly was disarmed. What had been right was now wrong – I couldn't even write. I described my hands as mutually*

37

*clumsy. What remained was a limp right hand and, for most tasks, the left just wasn't right. Doctors offered aggressive surgeries, tendon transfers and such, to cobble together a claw. I refused. I bought a condo and was determined to remodel it myself. When people tried to discourage me, pointing out that I was "unable." I replied, "I don't know. Either I'll get my right hand back, or learn to use the left, or some of each. No matter what, I'll win." This was in the early 90's. I invested in computers, cameras, and softwares, determined to reinvent myself in digital art. I typed with my good left, the right dead in my lap. I split the days between remodeling and the cameras and computers. It was slow. Eventually I was alternating hands. Often I spent more time dropping and picking up tools, than doing. I taught my lame right hand by talking to it. I persisted. I never gave up. I went on to become a best selling author in the area of digital graphics. A decade later, I had my right arm back. I proved the doctors wrong. To be disarmed is more than injury. It is a state of mind that allows malady to prevail.*

*~J.W.L.*

# Big-Fat-Bummers At Next Curve

In the first two chapters we told you what Apnea is, and described the three kinds of Apnea: Obstructive Sleep Apnea (OSA), Central Sleep Apnea (CSA) and Mixed Apnea. We also explained how the disease progressively undermines health and well-being. In this chapter we present current research on highly correlated afflictions, which should otherwise be known as Big-Fat-Bummers. We are going to talk about just how bad it can get. Apnea is a life wrecker, a health destroyer and a major Big-Fat-Bummer. For a young man in the prime of life, Apnea can land in your front seat and literally wither your life prospects. It can be like racing around a tight fast corner in a smoking red Maserati and ... meeting a Mack truck head-on. Feeding tube, anyone?

# What's a Highly Correlated Affliction?

By definition, a highly correlated affliction is a health problem or disease that has been found to appear with higher than normal statistical consistency among people who suffer from Apnea: people with Apnea usually suffer one or more of mankind's most unpleasant diseases. People just starting out with Apnea are likely to develop one or more of these other problems. Like a herd of maladies, these afflictions tear down and trample a person's health because of the manner in which interlocking stresses cross more and more systems of the body. Many of these diseases are precursors to Apnea, while others appear as a consequence, or outcome of Apnea. Often, the correlation works both ways. One of the most sobering things is how this list continues to grow as researchers find more health problems directly related to Apnea.

## Highly Correlated Afflictions

At present count, there are over thirty afflictions legitimately correlated with Apnea. We have endeavored to make our list comprehensive without duplication, but the real and critical point here is that a LOT can go wrong in association with Apnea.

Sometimes Apnea is the larger medical problem, while in other diagnoses it is a mere component of a larger set of problems. But it has been shown that attention to these problems always leads to an improvement in the symptoms in other areas. The reverse is also true; inattention to one of these health problems can result in a worsening of Apnea.

What is harder to explain is that the research also shows that, **for nearly every malady that can either worsen or improve Apnea, the opposite relationship is also true. Which is to say that treatment of the Apnea can help lead to improvement in such varied areas of ill-health as obesity, depression, vision problems or even learning problems.** If one were to attempt to explain these relationships to a child, you'd probably want to talk about a carousel. You can have Apnea alone or with any one of those horses, or even several; but you can also have just one of those other horses, ride it around going up-and-down until you find you've then got Apnea, too. And then many of those other horses will join your herd of ill health, too. It just goes round and round, bringing you further down. If only you had read the signs.

## 30+ Highly Correlated Afflictions
## Killers & Bummers

01.　Attention Deficit Hyperactivity Disorder (ADHD)

02.　Anxiety

03.　Asthma

04.　Blunt Force Trauma

05.　Brain Damage

06.　Bruxism (Teeth Grinding)

07.　Death

08.   Depression
09.   Diabetes
10.   Enuresis (Bed Wetting)
11.   Epilepsy
12.   Erectile Dysfunction
13.   Gastro Esophageal Reflux Disease (GERD)
14.   Glaucoma
15.   Hearing Loss
16.   Heart Attack
17.   Heart Disease
18.   Inflammation
19.   Jaw Problems
20.   Liver Disease
21.   Memory Loss
22.   Night Terrors
23.   Nocturia
24.   Obesity
25.   Ophthalmologic Conditions (in addition to glaucoma)
26.   Panic Attacks
27.   Periodic Limb Movement Disorder (PLMD)
28.   Restless Leg Syndrome
29.   Stroke
30.   Teeth grinding
31.   Testosterone Drop
32.   Thyroid Problems

# Killers and Bummers

In structuring this book, we decided that this chapter, Chapter Three, "Big-Fat-Bummers" should logically precede Chapter Four, "Killers." Why should Big-Fat-Bummers come before killers? Our reasoning is crucial to the entire project: **long-term Killer Afflictions are known to shorten your life**, but are often too abstract to garner immediate attention; the fact is that they invite denial. And usually, unless you have medical tests and a proper diagnosis, you won't really know that one of the killers has you.

## Pages Are Freedom, So Thumb Away!

One early reader commented that they'd have preferred it if we'd rearrange the book with these detailed excursions into medical maladies at the back. It was just too tedious and hard to read. Well, this is a book. It has pages. It is not a monorail or a trip on a space odyssey where the next stop is 25,000 miles. And there is no test on Monday. So, when you've read what is pertinent to you, turn to another part of the book. But do read on. Your life, or your wife, may depend on it.

Here's a good example: consider plaque that sometimes builds up in the coronary artery where it passes through the neck. A relatively unknown fact is that vibrations caused by heavy snoring can damage the inner lining, or endothelial wall, of the coronary artery, causing plaque build-up there. Without a body-scan, that plaque build-up continues out of sight and out of mind. No pain. No issue. "No worries mate." No. Not until a bit breaks off, travels up the artery to lodge in the brain, causing a stroke.

We'd say that's a killer. And if you were to survive the event, if you could talk, you'd say that you never knew it was coming.

By contrast, let's talk about GERD, commonly known as heartburn. Night after night, it takes no effort to be acutely aware of that burning in your throat, even though – at least, until now – you've had no awareness of the Apnea connection. But Apnea can and does cause GERD. This is a Big-Fat-Bummer. It's also something that, having your attention, may hopefully lead you to save your own life. Remember, your body wants to thrive.

## Two Birds, One Stone

Our title, "Sleep or Die," gets the direst message across, albeit harshly: Apnea Kills You. This chapter has more of a "Sleep or Live with a Big-Fat-Bummer" message. Since eighty percent of Apneacs are completely unaware that they have any form of Apnea – we hope to "kill two birds with one stone." And keep you alive.

### Bird One

Right now as you read this, you might realize that you have one of these "big-fat bummers," understand that you are touched by Apnea, and know that you need to learn more about the disease and take action; choose life. Because now is the time for you to save your life and also the quality of it, before you are saddled with a Killer Affliction.

### Bird Two

If you have Apnea and know that you really don't want any of the bummer afflictions, then this is the time to get motivated and overcome snoring and OSA before your health worsens and progresses to even worse things. **Hey, guys, it could even progress to something embarrassing, like ED (erectile** dysfunction). **We *are* going to talk about things that are a lot less fun than football. We aren't concerned about limp reviews. But you should be.** Because you could find yourself snoring, alone, with a tiny-limp-bummer, only to die later from a Killer Affliction.

# Highly Correlated Afflictions: The Big-Fat-Bummer Group

The oddest human behavior regarding health is our ability to ignore, repress, and deny our own disease. Especially when we know we are not well, but just don't feel it; at least, not in an acute way. Even if it's killing you. Out of sight, out of mind. Not so with these Big-Fat-Bummers. These will get your attention:

## ADHD

Attention Deficit Hyperactivity Disorder (ADHD) is generally a diagnosis for children. Yet because the two problems present with great similarity, **children are often misdiagnosed with ADHD when they are actually suffering with OSA**. Tiredness, lack of focus, and appearance of hyperactivity associated with ADHD can be caused by lack of sleep from OSA. Research now shows that as many as 30% of the children diagnosed of ADHD may instead have a sleep disorder. For both ADHD and OSA, the typical kid is as often skinny as fat, with big tonsils and adenoids, and a bed wetter. Bedwetting (enuresis) is especially symptomatic if the child is older than five, and has had a recurrence of bedwetting after having appeared to grow out of it. Even during waking hours, their large tonsils and adenoids may make it difficult for them to breathe through the nose. When children have trouble breathing in the daytime it is important to have a careful and thorough

44

evaluation. Symptoms may be from a simple condition like chronic congestion or allergies, or something worse like asthma, or, as we say, the loud killer, OSA.

Parents should not rest easy with an ill-defined diagnosis or explanation that their child, "just has problems breathing at night." **This really is too serious. Better to smother your child with love.** Often, children with OSA appear to sleep in contorted positions, arching their necks to open their throats, and they will get very sweaty from the increased work of their breathing.

Many children with Apnea have weight issues that may cause or contribute to their Apnea. While for other children, Apnea can adversely affect the production of growth hormone, which is secreted in sleep. Such an untimely disruption of a child's vital developmental process may, in turn, cause a failure to thrive, or even stunted growth. A misdiagnosis that leaves the OSA untreated – whether untreated because the child has OSA instead of ADHD or if untreated because the child suffers from both ADHD and OSA – can have long-term damaging effects to a child's health and development.

## Anxiety and Panic Attacks

A period of paused breath causes oxygen deprivation, meaning that there is not enough oxygen to fuel the brain. At the same time, the stoppage of breath causes a build-up of $CO_2$, which would normally be vented with breathing. Panic attacks are associated with a build-up of $CO_2$ in the blood stream.

**Oxygen deprivation from untreated OSA can eventually lead to brain damage in areas that are related to sleep**, thereby causing a vicious cycle of Apnea-induced oxygen deprivation leading to brain damage, which impairs breathing thereby exacerbating the Apnea and this appears to even further impair and damage the brain. Unfortunately, it gets worse. Researchers have shown that many of the same OSA processes that are injurious to the brain also play a part in the development of anxiety and panic attacks. Researchers at the University of Iowa have demonstrated that high levels of $CO_2$ cause an increase of brain acidity, which triggers a protein that is central to feelings of fear and anxiety. Additionally, there may also be a tie-in with night terrors, which are also thought to be triggered by a high build-up of $CO_2$.

## Asthma and GERD

Beyond the confusing similarity of the words, **the linkage between asthma and Apnea is complicated by the fact that both affect the breathing and the symptoms are most often experienced in the throat.** Additionally, both asthma and Apnea can be aggravated by gastro esophageal reflux disease (GERD).

For the purpose of this discussion, asthma is something doctors say, too often, that you are likely "born with" the predisposition to develop asthma (although it can also develop after exposure to high levels of airborne irritants), and that it is something you must deal with for the rest of your life. Throughout an asthmatic's lifetime there are many good choices for treatment and control. Asthma can be aggravated by GERD because the acid refluxed into the throat can be accidently inhaled at night, irritating the airways, causing them to constrict. Apnea is involved with GERD in two ways, one GERD-driven, and the other Apnea-driven.

### GERD-driven

With GERD-driven Apnea, digestive acid comes up the lower sphincter, and then makes it up the esophagus to irritate and constrict the upper air passage, obstructing breathing. Over time, the acid may irritate the esophagus or throat. In most cases, continuous irritation will cause a worsening of a patient's Apnea or asthma – or even both.

### Apnea-driven

With Apnea-driven GERD, the sleeper has an Apnea episode, and gasps for breath upon waking. This gasp creates a vacuum (negative pressure) drawing digestive acid up the esophagus, causing an episode of acid reflux, or after multiple episodes, GERD. The **inflammation and swelling that result from GERD worsens the Apnea sufferer's symptoms**. Similarly, the asthma sufferer is further harmed by the complication of GERD. So Apnea and acid reflux go hand in hand in a vicious cycle. The acid causes more inflammation and swelling, which leads to more obstruction. Large tonsils become more enlarged, leading to more severe breathing problems at night. Throat linings also become swollen from the acid, and the tongue becomes swollen, often leaving sores on both sides where the swelling rubbed the tongue onto the teeth.

## Brain Damage

The brain must have a constant, rich supply of oxygen. **Without oxygen, the brain stops functioning, and is <u>very</u> quickly damaged.** Because Apnea involves a lapse of breath, it usually means that the supply of oxygen is briefly, but repeatedly, cut off. This can result in slowly increasing damage to the brain that may be nearly undetectable. Damage will increase as the severity of Apnea worsens. A 2009 study showed that the connective fibers in the white matter of the brain are altered as a result of OSA; specific brain regions showed functional alterations, including areas that regulate memory and planning functions

# Brain Management

During Apnea episodes, the airway becomes blocked, hindering or stopping breathing and causing blood oxygen levels to drop and blood pressure to rise. Eventually the Apneac awakens and begins to breathe again, restoring "normal" blood oxygen and blood flow to the brain. As the primary organ of the body, the brain ordinarily regulates its own blood flow. But Apneacs suffer repeated surges and drops in blood pressure, blood flow, and blood oxygen level. Each night, these numerous episodes eventually reduce the brain's own ability to normalize and regulate such critical functions. This, in turn, increases the Apneac's exposure to all forms of disease.

**The brain-damage cycle accelerates Apnea.** Oxygen starvation may destroy connections within the brain. These damaged connections within the brain are a possible contributor to the Apnea itself. This means that **if you have untreated Apnea and it progresses to the point where your brain begins to suffer, then your Apnea may worsen. You may progress to CSA or Mixed Apnea** Plus, your untreated Apnea will cause other Apnea-related health risks, and is likely to spiral into any number of other highly correlated afflictions - many of which are shown to aggravate the underlying Apnea.

## Bruxism (Teeth Grinding)

To many, it's just common sense that sleepless nights are anxious nights and that anxious nights drive caffeine consumption. So does being tired during the day from poor sleep. It's also been clinically shown that both anxiety and teeth grinding are directly correlated with Apnea and that the presence of any one of these problems – whether it be Apna itself, or excess coffee drinking, or troubling anxiety – is a likely predictor for the development of the other two problems. This means that if you have Apnea, you might drink too much coffee, and you may grind your teeth at night. And in combination, these three problems will likely lead to more health problems over time. It's a vicious cycle of gasping, grinding and grogginess which lead to much too much caffeine, then anxious grinding insomnia, and then groggy again and then, yes, coffee.

## Depression

(Also see **Anxiety**)

Think of any movie where the character gets bumped off their flight, airport-stranded over night, and the scene opens with our bedraggled character not smiling, feeling depressed. Lack of sleep will do that to you. It's universal. But our research uncovers a correlation that's far more disturbing. It appears that while a lack of sleep can lead to depression, **Apnea is often the cause of depression itself**, which can lead to another vicious cycle of Apnea exacerbated by depression and consequently having a greater role in exacerbating the depression. Repeat. Repeat. Repeat. Thus, causing the patient even greater risk of further suffering from the other problems that appear as the patient's Apnea worsens. In a study of conditions resulting in death where depression was also involved, Apnea showed the highest co-morbidity and researchers found that patients diagnosed with Apnea had both the highest levels of depression and the highest use of antidepressants. The good news is that it doesn't have to be this way. The good news is that depression is not incurable and that Apnea need not worsen, much less lead to even more severe health problems. You do have options.

## Enuresis (Bed Wetting)

Please refer to **Attention Deficit Hyperactivity Disorder** for relevance to childhood Apnea. Also, see **Nocturia** for relevance of adult symptoms to Apnea.

## Epilepsy

People with epilepsy also have a high incidence of Obstructive Sleep Apnea (OSA). A University of Michigan study found that as many as one third of epilepsy patients also have OSA. The correlation of epilepsy with OSA has been shown to aggravate the course of both disorders. Sleep fragmentation in OSA not only increases drowsiness in epilepsy patients, it can even promote the occurrence of seizures. Conversely, epileptic seizures may also induce Apnea.

Much like Apneacs, epilepsy patients are often unaware of the seizures that occur while they sleep. They may suffer for years from daytime fatigue and concentration problems without ever knowing why. Sleep problems are a double-edged sword for epileptics. Epilepsy disturbs sleep and sleep deprivation aggravates epilepsy. Apneacs or not, achieving healthy sleep on a nightly basis is essential for people with epilepsy.

## Erectile Dysfunction

Fear of wilting reviews almost prevented us from including this section in the book. But we decided we should tell the whole truth. While erectile dysfunction may not come up often in polite conversation, there are enough ads on TV to clue everyone that this is a concern for many men – and their partners. Yet what is news is a surprisingly clear correlation between dissatisfactory romantic performance and OSA.

There are other obvious correlations, many of which reinforce the vicious cycle aspect of Apnea; erectile dysfunction may be a component of depression, which may appear as either a precursor or symptom of Apnea. One study of middle-aged obese men found that 63% had OSA. 5.6% also had diabetes, and 29% had a history of smoking. Statistical analysis revealed that men with erectile dysfunction are more than twice as likely to have OSA. It also correlated more severe erectile dysfunction with a greater likelihood of OSA. Another study documents a direct correlation of Apnea with ED: **of nearly 100 men suffering from ED (who had never been treated for Apnea), 75 experienced a remission in their ED symptoms after only one month of CPAP treatment**: hard wood had returned to the thickets of Eden.

## GERD

(See **Asthma**)

## Glaucoma

(See **Ophthalmological Conditions**)

## Hearing Loss

A new Taiwanese study suggests that people suffering from Obstructive Sleep Apnea are at a slightly greater risk of developing sudden hearing loss. A significant number of patients with OSA were found to be hemodynamically hyperviscosity positive, meaning that their blood is thicker and more prone to clog arteries. These patients were also shown to have a high rate of hearing loss. After 6 months of treatment with CPAP, hyperviscosity was normalized in over half the patients. Of those that normalized, a majority of patients were found to have restored normal hearing. One obvious conclusion of the study is the correlation of hearing loss with an underlying sleep-breathing disorder.

## Inflammation and Irritation

It makes common sense that inflammation or irritation of the throat and related areas would worsen both the symptoms and frequency of Apnea. But as with many other highly correlated maladies that accompany Apnea, inflammation and irritation are also partners in a vicious cycle. Apnea impairs the body's ability to process sugars (or, glucose metabolism) because repeated cycles of stop and go breathing, as well as the resulting sleep disturbance, lead to the release of excess stress hormones, primarily cortisol. Excess cortisol causes the accumulation of fat in the belly (specifically in the omentum), which in turn causes more inflammation thereby leading to a vicious cycle of worsening Apnea and worsening health.

Both tonsil problems and their common solution, tonsillectomy, can lead to inflammation and irritation. But can having tonsils removed make you fat? The common practice of childhood tonsillectomy, or removal of the tonsils, was studied. Researchers reviewed nine studies conducted between 1970 and 2009 with about 800 children up to age 18 who had their tonsils removed, with or without the removal of their adenoids. They found that **a year after surgery the average increase in BMI was around 7% among children who had their tonsils removed.** This procedure is also correlated with obesity because it can result in nerve damage, which changes the sensitivity to taste, causing the individual to both overeat. The overeating leads to obesity. Who knew having your tonsils removed could lead to obesity later?

## Jaw Problems

(See **Bruxism**)

## Liver Disease

A Johns Hopkins research team has shown that Obstructive Sleep Apnea (OSA) is implicated to the progression of liver disease – independent of obesity. They found that the severity of low levels of oxygen in the blood predicts the severity of insulin resistance and "may be implicated in the development of liver disease." Their report concludes that even without complications, severe obesity is the initial driver in the progression of liver disease, and that **chronic intermittent oxygen deprivation, as occurs with Apnea, acts as a second driver because oxygen deprivation stresses the livers of patients with severe obesity**, leading to further inflammation and progression of liver disease.

## Memory Loss

What were we talking about? Memory issues often accompany Apnea. Although no consistent correlation has been found between OSA severity and memory deficit, it is believed that Apnea may result in decreased memory and other thinking or cognitive abilities. **Among Apneacs, gray matter was reduced in areas of the brain that are linked to cognitive abilities and memory function that has been compromised.** Apneacs often exhibit a retrieval deficit of episodic memory but intact maintenance, recognition, and forgetfulness; they showed decreased overall performance in procedural memory, although pattern learning did occur; and impairment of specific working memory capabilities despite normal short-term memory. That's because the **oxygen deprivation resulting from Obstructive Sleep Apnea**

**(OSA) causes brain damage** that, in turn, leads to attention and memory problems. Researchers found that the gray matter of Apneacs is often reduced in areas of the brain linked to cognitive abilities, as well as deficits in the left cortex, which is associated with daytime sleepiness.

## Night Terrors, or Night Terror

Reduced airflow may trigger night terrors. **Apnea is implicated as a trigger of night terrors and sleepwalking.** The irregular breathing unnaturally disturbs slow wave sleep, triggering night terrors and other sleep disorders. This is true even with mild Apnea. It appears as if reduced airflow is the trigger for night terrors, much as if one were to awake while being choked, which of course sets off a panic. This would be especially true during REM sleep, because when the body goes into this deep sleep the sleeper is most vulnerable to episodes of night terror. The body's natural response to suffocation is to jump out of bed and wake; episodes of leaping terror defeat the body's system of freezing your muscles during dreaming. Among children who've had surgeries to improve their breathing, a reduction of night terrors has been an observed improvement.

# Pediatric Night Terrors and Nocturia

Children with night terrors are also likely to develop the parallel problem of bed wetting later. We know of one young boy who had terrible night terrors, which stopped for a while with an old wives trick of putting his feet into cool, not cold, water during an episode. Although much improved, neither the terrors nor the bedwetting stopped completely until his tonsils and adenoids were removed. Prior to that, however, the pediatricians had no recommendations. After some sleuthing on the web, particularly the Stanford Sleep Centers site, the child was brought to Stanford for consultation. The removal of his tonsils and adenoids was advised to open the airway. The results were phenomenal. So if your child (or you) suffers from night terrors or nocturia it would be worthwhile to learn more about sleep parasomnias and their connection to restricted air intake while sleeping.

Also among people with mild Apnea who have begun CPAP treatment, a reduction of night terrors occurs. This suggests that while Apnea may lead to night terrors, reduced airflow from other causes can also cause night terrors.

## Nocturia

Nocturia is simply the need to get up during the night to urinate. But it's often an indication of more. In addition to the link between Night Terrors and childhood bedwetting, researchers have also found a correlation between sleep disturbances and adult urinary problems. **Sleep problems often precede urologic conditions, such as urinary incontinence, lower urinary tract symptoms, and nocturia**. In cases where Apnea is also present, relief of the Obstructive Sleep Apnea often alleviates nocturia.

A 2003 poll of sleepers in America, found that 65% of adults age 55-84 report the need to get up to go to the bathroom a few nights a week or more, with 53% of those polled reporting the need to go every or almost every night. Short sleep duration among men and restless sleep among men and women is strongly associated with the incidence of lower urinary tract symptoms, with a frequency of 8 percent among men and 13 percent among women. These findings were peculiar in that those incidences of urinary incontinence and nocturia were associated with restless sleep among women but not men. Apnea-driven nocturia is more likely to be found in women, while age is said to be a factor, too.

Why would decreased sleep lead to increase of nocturia? Researchers found that the percentage of rapid eye movement sleep time correlates inversely with nocturic frequency. Apnea reduces REM sleep, so it's easy to connect the dots. But Nocturia is often a symptom of other serious medical conditions including urological infection, a tumor of the bladder or prostate, bladder prolapse, as well as disorders affecting sphincter control. Nocturia is common among people with heart failure, liver failure, and diabetes. If you have the symptoms, it's worth your while to rule those out.

## Ophthalmologic Conditions

### Floppy Eyelid Syndrome

Floppy eyelid syndrome is so named because in this syndrome, the eyelids turn inside out spontaneously during sleep, causing irritation. Excessive watering, stickiness, discomfort and blurred vision: while not a serious medical problem, it may indicate that the patient has OSA, which, as this book demonstrates, often leads to other more significant health problems.

### Glaucoma

Glaucoma is an eye disorder in which the optic nerve suffers damage, permanently damaging vision in the affected eye(s). Glaucoma is the second most common cause of blindness and irreversible blindness; untreated glaucoma progresses to complete blindness. It is often, but not always, associated with increased pressure of the fluid in the eye (aqueous humour).

OSA has been shown to be a likely contributor to at least two forms of glaucoma because it causes profound changes in oxygenation, circulatory hemodynamics, and inflammatory factors. All of these can influence optic nerve integrity and pressure within the eye as well. The two forms of glaucoma linked to Apnea are primary open-angle glaucoma, or POAG, and normal-tension glaucoma, or NTG. For both types, the **severity of the glaucoma correlates directly with the number and duration of Apnea episodes**.

### *Nonarteritic Anterior Ischemic Optic Neuropathy (NAION):*

There is a high prevalence (89%) of SAS, a form of Obstructive Sleep Apnea (OSA) among patients stricken with NAION, which is the occurrence of sudden painless vision loss in one eye, usually noticed on awakening, often causing irreversible vision loss.

Experts in the field of neuro-ophthalmology agree: the two main risk factors for NAION are (1) minor aberrations in the shape of the optic disc and (2) cardiovascular risks, specifically diabetes, hypertension and high levels of cholesterol. While these factors may predispose a patient to develop NAION, what is more significant is that the most common precipitating factor is a marked fall of blood pressure during sleep (nocturnal arterial hypotension).

This explains why most patients discover visual loss on first waking. Apnea, which also adversely impacts blood pressure, amplified by the vascular risk factors, leads to ischemia (poor blood supply) of a portion of the optic disc, which then swells. Among those with what is called a "crowded optic disc," **this condition results in nightly cycles of compression and ischemia leading, finally, to sudden blindness.**

## Panic Attacks

(See **Anxiety**)

## Periodic Limb Movement Disorder (PLMD)

Periodic limb movement disorder (PLMD) is a sleep problem where the patient's limbs move involuntarily during sleep, causing symptoms or problems related to those movements. Not be confused with restless leg syndrome (RLS), PLMD is involuntary, with the patient often completely unaware of these movements. (RLS occurs while awake as well as when asleep, and when awake, there is a voluntary response to an uncomfortable feeling in the legs.) **Symptoms of PLMD are excessive daytime sleepiness (EDS); falling asleep during the day, trouble falling asleep at night, and difficulty staying asleep throughout the night. These symptoms can be worsened if Apnea is also present.**

## Testosterone Drop

**Apnea is also related to a decrease in the production of testosterone, the primary male hormone.** Researchers at Teknion Israel Institute of Technology found that male patients suffering from OSA (Obstructive Sleep Apnea) produce lower levels of testosterone and have a corresponding reduction in libido and sexual activity. Their findings suggest that male OSA is associated with dysfunction of the pituitary-gonadal axis, involving luteinizing hormone (LH). They further correlate LH – testosterone profiles and the severity of OSA to suggest that sleep fragmentation and hypoxia as well as the degree of both obesity and aging are related to decreased testosterone. Yet there are conflicting views on the advisability of testosterone augmentation for Apnea sufferers.

# Testosterone and Apnea

When exploring treatment of an Apnea-related drop in testosterone, considering all risks, it is found that lean body mass, and not testosterone augmentation, is the first, if not the preferred solution to bettering both Apnea and testosterone drive. In fact, some studies have indicated that testosterone augmentation worsens Apnea and may even be dangerous.

## Thyroid Problems

Hypo-thyroidism occurs when the thyroid gland doesn't make enough thyroid hormone, causing the body to slow down. Symptoms include thin, brittle hair or fingernails, sensitivity to cold, constipation, depression, fatigue, heavier menstrual periods, joint or muscle pain, paleness or dry skin, weakness and weight gain. For most hypo-thyroid sufferers, unintentional weight gain is an inevitable consequence; that in turn, worsens the Apneac's symptoms. Studies show a direct correlation between increased weight and a jump in the patient's Apnea score, or AHI index. **Hypo-thyroidism aggravates Apnea, because when an Apneac gains in weight, especially in the neck, that weight gain directly correlates to a worsening of the Apnea.** When hypo-thyroidism is treated and if the patient Neck Circumference (NC) becomes smaller, the thyroid problem no longer factors in the patient's degree of Apnea.

Yet there are other, more complicated and troubling linkages between OSA and hypo-thyroidism. Sometimes, in unusual cases, an underactive thyroid is accompanied by an enlarged tongue, which is also highly correlated with Apnea. In this case, the tongue swells and becomes thicker and "scalloping" of the tongue occurs. Simply put, the enlarged tongue is pressing against the teeth and has nowhere to go. During sleep, when the tongue falls back into the air passage, it can either block breathing entirely or result in reduced airflow thereby causing Apnea episodes or hypopnea. But the most troubling linkage between Apnea and hypo-thyroidism is even more sinister: since both maladies are common, each occurring in about 2% of the North American population, they are often confused because they have common symptoms of obesity, fatigue, decreased libido, depressed mood, and impaired concentration. This presents a dangerous opportunity for a missed diagnosis of hypo-thyroidism, with dire long-term consequences for the undiagnosed patient.

# There Is No Final Word

With Big-Fat-Bummers, there is no end to the complications and travails that can land in your life. Like the proverbial old folks who just can't stop talking about their health problems, once you land in this terrain, you'll never run out of things to complain about. But is that where you want your life to lead? If not, choose differently. **Learn to read the signs**. For while these afflictions have multiple causes and effects, one agreed up on fact is that they are uncomfortable, unsettling, warning signs in the road.

Yes, these afflictions are often slow to progress, but they should not be ignored. Read on and get your own healing going.

# CHAPTER 4:
# Accessory to Murder

## *Angst*

*Being a responsible sort, I decided to use a CPAP machine after recognizing my surgery was not effective. So, Peter the CEO of one of the most successful CPAP manufacturers, offered me the chance to obtain one from his corporate lab. After getting it fitted, I headed home, put it on the bedside and tried it on. All was well.*

*Except one thing! I felt compelled to hide it during the day. It looked so medieval and so much like I was on my last legs, that I did not like to look at it nor did I want anyone to get the wrong idea. I am not even sure what that idea was, but it was a struggle to accept the CPAP.*

*Then one day, my angst and embarrassment shifted to embracement. I now view it as a technology that is saving me from the punishing evil OSA doles out. It's like a computer. I like to upgrade it. Regularly, I meet fellow Apneacs, who tell me they have had the same machine for ten years. How crazy is that? The level of improvement is amazing. Just think; the iPhone did not exist ten years ago. So now, I tell anyone who will listen "Go all in" with your treatment. Embrace and overcome.*

*~W.E.H*

# Apnea: Accomplished Accomplice to Killers

In the previous chapter, we talked about how bad it can get when Apnea is working its fiendish way, calling up one or more afflictions to join it in the degeneration of your body, your family, your life. Admittedly, that was rather dark. But in this chapter were going to talk about the darkest side, the ways in which Apnea can kill you.

That's right. We say that Apnea is an accessory to murder, a co-conspirator: because that's how we would best understand Apnea today if it were a person. Apnea hangs with the baddest killers.

That said, do remember, p-l-e-a-s-e: this is a book, not a monorail with no stops for the next 2,000 miles. The advantage of a book is that pages can be turned, and you can choose to turn to the next chapter or section. You won't hurt our feelings. Honestly. We won't even know. We don't have the technology for that. Yet.

So until that day, we'll continue to advise our readers to skip stuff that's not relevant to them, or what they think is not relevant. It may be relevant later, and then you'll know to look back to the parts you skipped in this book. Alrighty then. Read what you can stomach.

## Dead End Road

We now know that untreated Apnea drives killer diseases in the body. Twenty years ago little was known about the profound downstream effects of Apnea. No longer. The correlations between heart disease and OSA, between diabetes and OSA are now understood. Apnea is behind the wheel, driving both diseases. Apnea is a dead end. As shown in the following table, data from Centers for Disease Control and Prevention (CDC) and the National Center for Health Statistics (NCHS) heart disease and diabetes are among the biggest contemporary killers:

### Biggest Contemporary Killers
### Ranked By Number of Deaths
### (Centers for Disease Control and Prevention
### & National Center for Health Statistics)

01. Diseases of heart

02. Malignant neoplasms (cancers)

03. Chronic lower respiratory diseases

04. Cerebrovascular diseases (brain blood supply)

05. Accidents (unintentional injuries)

06. Alzheimer's disease

07. Diabetes mellitus

08. Influenza and pneumonia

09. Nephritis, nephrotic syndrome & nephrosis (kidneys)

10. Intentional self-harm (suicide)

11. Septicemia (blood poisoning)

12. Chronic liver disease & cirrhosis

13. Hypertension & hypertensive renal disease (high blood pressure)

14. Parkinson's disease

15. Assault (homicide)

These high-profile killer afflictions are too often found in the company of Apnea. Other culprits of high statistical dread, such as Cerebrovascular (Heart) Diseases, also appear in the Apnea rap sheets of highly correlated killers, which are detailed here in the following sections of this chapter.

# Highly Correlated Killers

## Blunt Force Trauma

Statistically, most Blunt Force Trauma is from auto accidents. The good news is that this is because there are more people driving cars than there are axe murderers. Though the way some people drive might lead you to wonder, or at least roll up your window. The bad news is that, if you are an Apneac, and you are driving, you really should roll all the windows down.

**That's because as an Apneac behind the wheel, you are the worst threat to your own life and limb.**

In fact, twenty years ago, when we knew far less about the afflictions that accompany Apnea; the gravest danger about which Apnea patients were commonly warned was increased risk of falling asleep at the wheel of an automobile. At the time, it was also one of the most compelling reasons for treatment.

Although modern medical science now recognizes more reasons to test for and treat Apnea, it's still relevant to be concerned about sleep-deprived driving. According to a recent study, patients with moderate to severe Apnea have a fifteen-fold greater risk of motor vehicle accidents. A study of truckers with sleep-disordered breathing revealed that they have double the accidents per mile.

# I Can't Drive BMI 35!

When I heard the Federal Motor Carriers Safety Administration (FMCSA) has Apnea regulations in the works to screen drivers for Apnea, my ears perked up. A primary screening tool will be Body Mass Index (BMI); if a driver's BMI is greater than 35, then additional tests will be required to rule out Apnea.

Immediately, my own variation of Sammy Hagar's 1984 song, "I *Can't Drive 55*" played in my head.

> *Go on; write me up for being fat.*
> *Post my face: Wanted, dead or alive.*
> *Yeah, take my license 'n jive like that,*
> *I can't drive... BMI 35.*

Professional transportation workers, like truck drivers, have an especially difficult challenge. The nature of their work is sedentary and healthy eating is always complicated. But healthy eating while on the road and keeping up with the demands of the job is even more challenging.

But Apnea causes sleepy drivers, and that's more than just a health concern, it's dangerous for everyone on the road. Even pedestrians. Proposed FMCSA regulations will cast a wide net over those driving trucks and yank likely Apneacs into the medical system.

FMCSA pending-regulations focus on the same predictors as researched in this book:

- ✓ Drivers with a Body Mass Index (BMI) of 35 or greater.

- ✓ Male drivers with a neck size of 17 inches or greater.

- ✓ Female drivers with a neck size of 15.5 inches or greater.

- ✓ Male and female drivers with a BMI of over 28 who have had a crash.

- ✓ Drivers with a family history of Apnea.

- ✓ Drivers with a small jaw.

If a driver has any of these predictors, they will be required to have further tests to rule out Apnea. And if Apnea has them, they'll be required to treat the Apnea and show consistent compliance to keep their jobs.

No No No I can't drive, I CAN'T DRIVE BMI 35, I can't drive, I can't drive, I CAN'T DRIVE BMI 35! I CAN'T DRIVE BMI 35... **unless** I get treatment!

As of this writing, six US states require physicians to report patients who drive impaired, including those who may be chronically sleep-deprived. Another 25 states permit physicians the discretion to violate patient confidentiality in order to report sleep-deprived drivers. **Nationwide, crashes involving drowsiness or fatigue number over 100,000 annually, accounting for 1,500 fatalities and 71,000 injuries.**

Nationwide, many motor carriers have begun screening for and treating Apnea in the population of commercial drivers, with improved accident statistics. Recent legislation will soon force all motor carriers (and others whose workforce presents a risk to the public) to screen for Apnea.

As motor vehicle accident statistics rack up, it's only logical to expect that OSA will become a bigger deal – not only for driving but also for occupations and activities that involve the operation of vehicles and machinery. And occupational screening is likely to include a closer examination of applicants' medical records for afflictions highly correlated with Apnea, such as diabetes, which if uncontrolled can lead to unconsciousness or even a coma.

## Diabetes

Diabetes is a killer. Research shows that Apnea is a prevalent and important determinant of insulin resistance, glucose intolerance, and the likelihood of Type 2 Diabetes. As we know, Apnea can ruin sleep for years. Over a period of six years, individuals who slept less than six hours a night were found more likely to develop abnormal blood sugar levels, a precursor to Type 2 Diabetes.

In short, **Apnea has been shown to be a factor in the development of insulin resistance, glucose intolerance, and Type 2 Diabetes**. These are serious risks because diabetes is a killer. Diabetes affects more than 20 million Americans; 95% of them have Type 2, and over 40 million Americans have pre-diabetes, known as early Type 2 Diabetes.

### *Three Types of Diabetes*

- ✓ **Type 1 Diabetes:** Although usually diagnosed in childhood, many patients are diagnosed when they are older than age 20. Although the exact cause remains unknown, current science seems to concur that the Type 1 Diabetes patient's own immune system mistakenly destroys the cells in the pancreas that make insulin, the hormone that controls the level of blood sugar in the body. So the body makes little or no insulin. Life depends on daily injections of insulin. Research continues in several areas, including genetics, viruses, and autoimmune problems which may play a role.

- ✓ **Type 2 Diabetes:** This is the most common form of diabetes. Until recently, it occurred mostly among adults, but young people are increasingly being diagnosed with the disease. Again, the exact causes remain unknown.

Type 2 Diabetes is usually brought on by obesity and inactivity in people who have a genetic predisposition to develop the disease when they gain weight. It is thought that the "modern" diet may play a large factor in the shifting demographics of this disease. With Type 2 Diabetes, the result is that the patients' pancreas doesn't make enough insulin to keep blood glucose levels normal, often because the body does not respond well anymore to insulin – a condition called insulin resistance. Although a serious condition, many people with Type 2 Diabetes don't know they have it.

Initial treatment includes dietary changes, exercise and oral medicines, but many people eventually need insulin. In yet another vicious cycle which may ultimately include Apnea, incidence of Type 2 Diabetes is rising across all populations due to increasing obesity and failure to exercise – and both obesity and loss of muscle tone due to lack of exercise are shown to be highly correlated with Apnea.

✓ **Gestational Diabetes:** Occurring only among women who do not have diabetes, Gestational Diabetes is the abnormal increase of blood glucose that may develop during pregnancy. Women with Gestational Diabetes are at high risk for Type 2 Diabetes and cardiovascular disease later in life, both of which are also highly correlated with OSA.

Diabetes is a killer. Diabetes is known to correlate not only with Apnea, but is also highly correlated with many of Apnea's other "life" partners; poor diet, obesity, loss of muscle tone, cardiovascular disease, and death.

## Heart Disease

### Arrhythmias

Unlike other heart disease patients for whom sudden death tends to occur within a few hours after waking up, research shows that people with Apnea are more likely to suddenly die from arrhythmia during sleep. One form of arrhythmia, atrial fibrillation, is often lethal and otherwise complicates the management of advanced heart disease. It's been shown that all three types of Apnea – OSA, CSA, and Mixed Apnea – correlate directly with specific arrhythmias:

✓ OSA, Obstructive Sleep Apnea, is known to increase an Apneac's odds of developing ventricular arrhythmias.

✓ Apneacs with CSA, or Central Sleep Apnea, are more likely to suffer heart failure from ventricular fibrillation.

✓ All Apneacs are at increased odds of developing AF, or atrial fibrillation.

Untreated, **Apneacs are far more likely to suffer a ventricular arrhythmic arrhythmia or ventricular fibrillation event and will often die of brain or heart damage**. "Lucky" survivors often need surgery for an implant cardiac defibrillator (ICD), further complicating the management of their heart disease.

## Types of Cardiac Arrhythmia

Arrhythmias are life-threatening because they severely decrease the heart's ability to pump blood throughout the body. When an arrhythmia continues for more than a few seconds, blood circulation stops, and organ or brain damage may occur within minutes. Life-threatening arrhythmias include ventricular tachycardia and ventricular fibrillation. Arrhythmias are named to describe where they occur in the heart (atria or ventricles) and by what happens to the heart's rhythm when they occur.

When the heartbeat is accelerated to more than 100 beats per minute it is a tachycardia, while bradycardia occurs when the heartbeat slows to less than 60 beats per minute.

Arrhythmias that start in the atria are called atrial or supraventricular (above the ventricles) arrhythmias. Ventricular arrhythmias begin in the ventricles and are very serious because they are usually caused by heart disease.

## *Hypertension (High Blood Pressure) and Stroke*

Researchers have found that **adults with severe Apnea were more than twice as likely to have hypertension** (high blood pressure), while moderate Apneacs also had increased risk for high blood pressure. These findings held true even when the effects of obesity were factored into the study. Often, hypertension causes damage to the cardiovascular walls, which the body repairs with cholesterol. Cholesterol forms a plaque that can be dislodged, thereby reducing or even stopping the flow of blood to the brain. This exposes Apneacs to an even greater probability for stroke-related events.

## Heart Attack

Across the board, **untreated Apnea is associated with increased risk of high blood pressure, heart attack, irregular heartbeats, heart failure, and death**. The body is a complicated organism and it's hard to pinpoint when one thing has caused another, but it's clear that Apnea and heart events are related, like evil cousins out to do a body harm.

# Relief is Not Healed

Although the symptoms of Apnea may be eased or even healed with a combination of TOOLs, Apneacs experiencing improvement through exercise and/or the information and ideas in this book should most definitely continue supervised medical treatment for any form of heart disease, most especially stroke. Relief from Apnea is not necessarily a sign that one is healed of any associated or correlated condition.

## Stroke, or Cerebrovascular Accident (CVA)

Stroke is the leading cause of serious long-term disability and the third leading cause of death in the United States; it cripples over half a million people and kills another 150,000 more annually. **People with Apnea are more likely to suffer strokes and die in their sleep.** For too long, Apnea has been an unrecognized contributor to suffering and death from strokes.

According to the National Institutes of Health (NIH), Apnea more than doubles the risk of stroke in men. A comparison of coronary Apneacs to coronary patients without Apnea showed the Apneacs are 3 times more likely to suffer a stroke.

Independent of other risk factors, **heavy snoring significantly increases the risk of carotid atherosclerosis, or carotid artery disease, which occurs when cholesterol accumulates into plaques in one or both of the carotid arteries**, located on either side of the neck. Eventually this narrowing limits or blocks the supply of blood to the brain, leading to stroke or mini-stroke. TIA (transient ischemic attack) is the medical term for a reversible "mini-stroke."

## Fat Dominoes

**What is Fat?** Fat is a tissue referred to as "adipose" and is the body's method of storing energy. Think of it as long-term storage. Much like the hard drive of a computer. Now, imagine if you had a computer with more than one hard drive. The body has a similar situation and stores this long-term energy, or fat, in different locations around the body.

**Location, Location, and Location:** Visceral fat is located within the abdominal wall for easy energy accessibility. It's close to the organs and can be converted quickly when needed. Epicardial fat is a particular form of visceral fat stored around the heart. Subcutaneous fat is stored under the skin, much like having a hard drive outside a computer but still connected.

**Fat by Color:** Fat comes in two colors: white and brown. White fat is common and well understood. Brown fat is rare and also less understood.

72

**White Fat:** White fat is stored in a semi-liquid state made up of triglycerides and cholesterol ester. White fat cells secrete proteins as adipokines: such as resistin, adiponectin, and leptin. Thirty pounds of fat in a human represents around 30 billion fat cells. When we gain weight as an adult, fat cells increase in size four times before dividing. Once divided, the overall number of fat cells increases.

**Brown Fat:** Brown fat has a different structure and shape, as well as a large number of iron-containing mitochondria, responsible for giving it a brown color. Brown fat has more circulation via capillaries since it has more need for oxygen. Newborn babies have more brown fat than adults. Brown fat can burn fast, creating heat to protect the newborn from getting cold. According to a 2012 New York Times story, research on brown fat's role in adults is literally on fire. It appears that brown fat may burn white fat. It also appears that staying cold creates brown fat, as may exercise. This is all of great interest because the more brown fat burns white fat, the more weight loss. Years ago, it was theorized that adults had no use for brown fat and it disappeared with maturity. Now, it's big. Not the amount of brown fat – that's still tiny, at less than an ounce on the entire body. But it's big because it may hold clues to combat obesity.

## Obesity

Most of us know that obesity is on the rise, like an evil tide, and is hard on the body. One surprising number: over 60 percent of all Americans are either overweight or obese. Just look around: we are drowning in a fat tsunami.

Obesity is especially rough on Apneacs. Fatty tissue surrounding the neck pushes on the airway, causing the wall to bulge inward; the degree of collapse has been shown to be proportional to the amount of tissue. What does this mean? **If a person develops Apnea after gaining an excess twenty pounds and develops an Apnea-Hypopnea Index of 10, gaining an additional twenty pounds will very likely increase the AHI, particularly if the weight gain deposits additional tissue in the neck region.** Neck fat is subcutaneous. When you lose weight, subcutaneous fat ("white fat") tends to decrease evenly throughout the body. This is good for improving the plumbing in the neck. Less fat around the neck results in more breathing room.

### Obesity and Omentum's Dire Momentum

Many types of fat exist in the human body: subcutaneous fat under the skin, blood fats, and omentum fat found in the belly. But what's brown fat? According to Drs. Roizen and Oz in their book, *"You On A Diet: the Owner's Manual for Waist Management,"* the fat of the omentum is dangerous <u>when in excess</u>. The omentum is the belly fat that hangs underneath the stomach muscle, surrounding the gut. (Don't confuse the omentum with a deposit of subcutaneous tummy fat; the omentum is located deeper in the abdomen, and is connected to the stomach.) This fat is ready energy because it is located close to the major organs and is quickly accessible to the liver. But when a person becomes obese, the omentum is often unusually enlarged with fat.

## Weight Worsens

A study of nearly 700 randomly selected Wisconsin residents showed a direct relationship between weight gain and worsening Apnea. The research showed that **a 10% increase in weight predicts a 6-fold increase in the odds of developing moderate-to-severe Apnea**. Relative to an Apneac's stable weight, a 10% weight gain predicts 32% increase in the Apnea-Hypopnea Index (AHI); while a 10% weight loss led to a 26% decrease in AHI.

The omentum's intersection with Apnea is complex. But to keep things simple, it's important to recognize that there are multiple mechanisms by which Apnea may impair glucose metabolism: just three are the repetitive cycles of hypoxemia and re-oxygenation, the related sleep fragmentation, and the resulting release of hormones such as cortisol which lead to the accumulation of fat in the omentum. This fat in the omentum initiates an inflammatory process that irritates the arteries, thereby putting the patient at increased risk for heart disease.

In addition to the problems associated with hormones such as cortisol, another hormone that is disrupted by the omentum is Adiponectin, a stress and inflammation-reducing chemical. Simply put, the basic relationship is this: less body fat means that you have more Adiponectin. Related to hunger hormones, Adiponectin helps muscles turn fat into energy and suppresses appetite. Omentum fat suppresses Adiponectin, which impacts the production of another hormone, Leptin, which shuts off hunger and stimulates the body to burn more calories. Thus, excess omentum fat leads to a cycle of disruption whereby the body/mind is not told to stop eating, which in turn feeds greater obesity. Finally, omentum also sucks insulin out of the blood stream. This outcome is unhelpful because the absence of insulin causes blood sugar to rise. When blood sugar goes up, insulin production needs to go up to counterbalance the sugar levels. It is thought that the repetition of this cycle, over and over, causes insulin resistance, which often leads to diabetes.

So here's the bottom line on omentum: obesity is complex. The complexity of obesity is compounded by the manner in which excess fat is often stored in the omentum, which in turn sets off a series of reactions that can spiral out of control, leading to greater obesity, diabetes, heart disease and, of course, worsening Apnea.

# Killer Conclusion?

Correlations are undeniable. Death doesn't bargain. Like a death sentence, the conclusions of this chapter are that short. That's the grave analysis.

So, is it flowers, or donations to your favorite charity? Or, are you going to get up now and get serious about getting healthy? Remember, your body wants to thrive.

Your friends and family want you to thrive, too. Probably, they are even depending on you.

To thrive. Not just survive.

So here's hope: Read on. Get your game on.

# CHAPTER 5:
# Predictors of Apnea

## *Stud Verses Dud*

*I look back at the versions of denial I experienced. They were classic and deep. The first assumption was that my partner would not be interested in sleeping in the same room with me if I have an air pump and mask strapped to my face. It's not the most delightful sound to my spouse, but she prefers the pump sounds to my snoring and gasping for breath twenty times an hour. I meet many spouses and partners who will not sleep in the same room unless their Apneac partner wears their treatment device. I used to collect stories of second-hand snorers and downwind Apneacs who had murdered their snoring, sleep-depriving, untreated Apneac partner, but then I thought I had better not tempt fate.*

*~W.E.H.*

## Trouble Likes Company

It should be in the headlines. **News flash: Evil Twins Predicted to Hang out Together.** Why in the headlines? Because Apnea and obesity are predictors of each other. Evil twins, if you will.

Where one is present, the other can't be too far behind. This means that if you have Apnea, you are likely to become obese. If you are obese, you probably already have Apnea or else are likely to develop it. So it goes with each of the highly correlated afflictions.

## Got Apnea?

In the last two chapters we hope to have seriously bummed you out. We can't help you to heal yourself unless you understand just how serious Apnea can be: and that it's not just serious for you, it impacts everyone around you. **There are more than thirty ways that Apnea can gang up with other villains to trounce you**.

Repeat: Got Apnea? Then you are likely to suffer from one or more of those afflictions. Like delinquents piled in an old hearse, they gang up in twos and threes, four or more, to make your health worse. And worse. And they do it with a deadly, life-sucking synergy.

## Predictors

Stepping down off our soapbox now, in this chapter we talk about what we call Predictors of Apnea. Our word, "predict," comes from Latin with the meaning, "to tell ahead of time." So, when someone can predict the future it means that they can tell what's going to happen before it happens. It's that simple. It's a finely honed ability that comes from observing the associations between real-life conditions.

We say that **a health predictor is a symptom or a change in your body telling you that something else may happen soon**. Often, such a predictor is really a separate disease. But when we look at patterns of disease in individuals and in populations, we can see that one health problem, malady or disease often increases our vulnerability to other diseases and health problems. In the same way that the common cold, when not cared for or even ignored, can lead to a life-threatening bronchitis or pneumonia, so too can other ailments lead and point to a future with Apnea. We call such ailments predictors.

Most, if not all, predictors of Apnea can also appear simultaneously or subsequent to the advent of Apnea. Which begins to make Apnea look like the leader in a downward spiral of ill health. This means that **ailments that are predictors and companion ailments to Apnea, as well as Apnea itself, are also likely yet to be suffered when initial symptoms go unnoticed or unheeded**. Ignoring symptoms such as GERD and obesity is like motoring down a road and seeing the signs that say quite clearly and in large letters, "danger ahead, watch for falling oxygen saturation levels." The key point here being that the early symptom comes before an even worse health problem and that this later worse health problem might have been easily controlled, much earlier on, by looking into that initial earlier symptom.

## I Simply Deny, Do I?

"Don't deny it, you know you are the first to deny it," is what she always says.

One of the fascinating things about Apnea is that the Apneac, the person who is suffering is usually, seemingly, the last to know. Well, "know" may be the wrong description.

How about the last to believe it is happening?

Well, maybe not "believe."

How about, "get-it-through-their-thick-head" that everyone around them (those unruly second-hand snorers and down-wind Apneacs), that, well, they just aren't making it up?

That sounds about right.

Because THE biggest predictor of Apnea is "partner observed cessation of breathing." It is that simple. But can <u>you</u> believe it?

## Denial

You might ask, "Why do so many Apneacs go without treatment until it's too late?" You could also ask, "What is the first crucial hurdle for any Apneac who wants to heal, get better, or at the very least, not get any worse?" The answer to these questions, quite simply, is both: "Denial." And also, "Overcoming denial."

Denial. **It's bigger than the world's longest river; a river travelled with eyes closed from the banks of health, your greatest wealth, to the mouth of death. Denial.**

Denial partners well with Apnea because Apnea skulks around when your guard is down, because vigilance is turned way down while we are sleeping, or at least trying to sleep. No wonder the Apneac is unaware of the problem. Even 10 seconds after being awakened by a partner, the typical Apneac completely denies snoring. Apneacs almost uniformly require irrefutable proof of snoring and cessation of breathing. So, get over the first hurdle and seek proof. The truth will set you free ... and save your health, your marriage, your quality of life.

### TOOL Makers

One of the things that separate humankind from the other animals is our ability to make and use TOOLs. We make and use TOOLs to get things done and to solve problems. Apnea is a problem. Our purpose in writing this book is to define the problem, and then to offer the TOOLs to solve it. **The first TOOL is a choice that every Apneac can make over the course of their disease: attack denial**. This TOOL isn't simple, but it is an on-off switch, a toggle, a sharp decision to cut the denial.

If you are an Apneac and aren't ready to make that decision, then (unless you like really scary stories full of suffering and lingering death) this book is worthless to you. But for the Apneac who has taken this first TOOL in hand, for the Apneac now moving out of denial, ready to accept that he or she has a disease called Apnea, **we offer a TOOLbox to overcome your evil disease, Apnea**. In the following chapters we will discuss the other TOOLs in detail. For now, though, let's continue to define the breadth of this health problem by examining the six predictors of Apnea.

# Six⁺ Predictors of Apnea

There are six broadly agreed upon predictors for the arrival of Apnea. It's widely noted that many of these predictors often appear long before Apnea presents. In 2010, three research groups conducted a novel statistical medical research study. The Department of Biostatistics and the Department of Epidemiology, both at Johns Hopkins Bloomberg School of Public Health, together with the Department of Preventive Medicine and Institute for Global Health at the University of Southern California, collaborated to plow through data on 5,000 patients and correlate it to Apnea. Beginning with a field of over forty potential predictors, the Johns Hopkins – USC study zeroed in on the top six predictors. They ranked these ailments according to the likelihood that they would lead to Apnea.

## Undiagnosed or Denied, Still Dead

In the patients with mild irregular heartbeat called ventricular premature contraction, more than 40 percent also have severe Apnea, and either don't realize it or just frankly deny it. While most people with this mild version of arrhythmia will be just fine, for some, Apneacs especially, it can worsen during the night and lead to a sudden death. You can deny your Apnea and still fail to wake up, having just died overnight.

We added one more predictor, which we liken to the zero point on a numeric scale. That predictor is denial of independently observed cessation of breathing. Here's our logic: **most, if not all, Apneacs learn of their disease from their sleeping partner**. (If you sleep alone, likely your roommates or neighbors down the street will eventually report to you of your dreadful snoring.) If you don't or won't believe the report, you're in denial. If you can't budge past that zero point – which is the first sign on the scale – then you are headed for more Apnea and worsening health.

As shown in the following table, there are seven predictors of Apnea: Denial of Third-party Observed Cessation of Breathing, Neck Circumference (NC), Body Mass Index (BMI), Age, Snoring Frequency, Waist Circumference, and Snoring Loudness.

### Seven Predictors of Apnea

00. Denial of Third-party Observed Cessation of Breathing

01. Neck Circumference

02. Body Mass Index

03. Age

04. Snoring Frequency

05. Waist Circumference

06. Snoring Loudness

# PREDICTOR ZERO:

## Denial of Third-Party Observed Cessation of Breathing

This is the bottom line. **If you're observed snoring heavily and then not breathing for multiple seconds up to a minute, repeatedly, you have some form of Apnea**. This is the quickest, easiest way to confirm that something's wrong. Do you believe them?

## Zero Has An Accomplice: Denial.

Don't let denial get in the way. While it is true that you shouldn't attempt to fix what is not broken, it's equally true that you can't correct what you don't know is broken. And if you won't admit something is broken, then you're in about the same fix as not knowing.

No real healing action is ever taken while the need for correction is denied. Remember, it is your own healing. Denial is the pivotal hindrance to opening the Apnea Avenger's TOOLbox. While this applies to all medicine and forms of health, including physical, mental and spiritual health, it is especially true with regards to the message of this book.

Any movement towards healing of Apnea requires that the Apneac's own denial be addressed. Additionally, if there is denial or misinformation from family, loved ones and friends, that too must be addressed. Otherwise, these six predictors are little more than a map to each and every Apneac's slow decline.

# Enter, Apnea Avengers!

Those who choose to open the Apnea Avenger's TOOLbox and move against their dreaded foe and its pantheon of dark dastardly accomplices, reported now to number 30 strong or more, will henceforth be anointed, Apnea Avenger!

# PREDICTOR ONE:

### Neck Circumference (or Neck Size) (NC)

Predictor One is pivotal for any healing of OSA. It's also pivotal to our understanding of the disease and how an Apneac might recover from it. As shown in the graph on the following page, Neck Circumference (NC) by far outperforms even its second best predictor by nearly double. Apnea Avengers take note!

In previous chapters we explored the prevalence of obesity among Apneacs and how it correlates with OSA. Nearly all doctors know, and all studies show that Neck Circumference (NC) is the top predictor and indicator of OSA (Obstructive Sleep Apnea). Also, **Neck Circumference is one of the simplest and most reliable methods to determine whether a person is clinically obese**. In the high correlation between OSA and obesity, Neck Circumference (NC) is both a diagnostic data point and predictor for both. It also accompanies most, if not all, of the other degenerative maladies that wreak their worsening power over the Apneac's life.

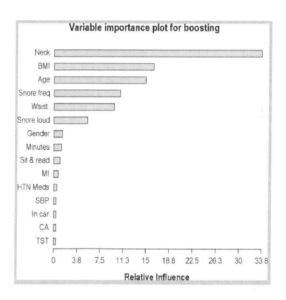

### Your Neck May Be Killing You

That's right, your neck may be killing you. Take a good look in the mirror. Get a measuring tape. Measure and record your neck size. As we will repeat and re-emphasize throughout this book, **nearly all of the healing TOOLs for Apnea are effective because they also work to reduce your neck size** or Neck Circumference (NC), which gives you, quite literally, breathing room.

## Weighing Genius

Calories-In is a HUGE factor in reducing Neck Circumference. Einstein himself reputedly stated in a famous 1939 speech to the Physics Department at Princeton, "You have to exercise for a week to work off the thigh fat from a single Snickers." He was right about that, too. It takes a lot of work to burn off a Snickers bar. So if you are trying to lose weight and you are eating candy, even with exercise you're probably going maintain or even gain weight. Two Hershey's Kisses require a half-mile walk to zero out those chocolate calories. King-size Snickers? That's 5 miles.

## Snorting and Snoring: What is Snoring?

We all know what pigs do. They snort. Snort, snort, snort again. Perhaps a snort is just a daytime snore. Not really. The structures involved in snoring are the uvula and soft palate. (The uvula is the floppy thing dangling at the back of your throat while the soft palate consists of the soft curtains around the uvula.) In humans, snoring results when an irregular airflow is caused by a blockage of the air passage in or around the uvula and soft palate.

## Air Traffic Constriction

Airway restrictions leading to OSA compromise the airway at any of six sites, or six areas. These can be partial or major blockages occurring alone or in myriad combinations. Starting at the tip of the nose and continuing all the way down to the lungs, the six constricted airway areas are: deviated or blocked nasal septum; large swollen nasal turbinates; uvula tissue; tongue size too big for its mouth box; weak, small-in-diameter or damaged pharyngeal throat muscles; and enlarged tonsils and adenoids.

### Constricted Airway Culprits

01.  Deviated or blocked nasal septum

02.  Large or swollen turbinates

03.  Uvula tissue

04.  Tongue size too big for cranial structure

05.  Weak, small or damaged pharyngeal throat muscles

06.  Enlarged tonsils and adenoids

# The Neti Pot

A neti pot (rhymes with spaghetti) is used for the purpose of personal hygiene to flush mucus from the nose and sinus. Originating in ancient India, this practice is also referred to as nasal irrigation, nasal lavage, or nasal douche, and can be an effective treatment for a wide range of sinus and nasal symptoms.

It's a simple technique that uses gravity and head positioning to pour a warm saline solution in one nostril and to let it run out through the other nostril, while keeping the mouth open to breathe. The saline solution is administered with a neti pot ("neti" is Sanskrit for "nasal cleansing"), which is commonly made of inexpensive plastic with a spout at one end and a handle on the opposite side, looking much like a small teapot.

While more advanced, electronic irrigation machines are also available; the common neti pot is usually sufficient for the purpose of maintaining a clean airway, and can be beneficial in treating for OSA because the nostrils are one of the six blockage points that lead to Apnea. *Care should be taken NOT to use ordinary tap water due to the rare possibility of lethal amoebic infection.* Neti pots and instructions for proper use, including recipes for saline solution, can be found online as well as at most reputable health food stores.

# PREDICTOR TWO:

## Body Mass Index (BMI)

Physicians rely upon BMI as a simple measure of fatness or thinness. The Johns Hopkins – USC statistical study cites BMI as the second most consistent predictor of Obstructive Sleep Apnea (OSA).

| BMI | Indication |
|---|---|
| Less than 20 | Underweight |
| 20-25 | Optimal weight |
| Over 25 | Overweight |
| Over 30 | Obese |
| Over 40 | Morbidly Obese |

The key point of BMI is that a high BMI number usually means too much fatty tissue for the body size. As pointed out with Neck

Circumference, fat in the wrong place, like the neck, reduces airflow. The most critical loss of breathing room occurs at night, when muscles relax and gravity flattens the horizontal throat.

## A Flawed Index

Unfortunately, the Body Mass Index is itself rather flawed. BMI is a calculation that attempts to arrive at a measure for the percentage of body fat in a person's body. But the calculation, which is based on a person's weight and height, was *developed for use in population studies and not for individual diagnosis.* Yet that is precisely how BMI is applied to the discussion of Apnea: a TOOL for population studies has been adopted for use in diagnosing individuals, so it is not precise.

### Understanding BMI

Despite its shortcomings, it's worthwhile to understand how BMI is read. The chart on the preceding page lists BMI indices in the left column, correlated with the general classification, ranging from underweight to morbidly obese, in the right column.

# PREDICTOR THREE:

## Age

As the graph on the following page demonstrates, statistics show that as an Apneac ages, their Apnea will usually get worse. At mid-life, one's Apnea is likely to be at its worst and then

89

gradually lessen as the person becomes more elderly. This trending of the disease itself, culled from clinical observations, warn us that Apnea will become epidemic as the baby boomer generation ages.

**Between the ages of 40 and 60, any problem with Apnea predicts a long steady decline into worsening health and complications from one or many of the highly correlated afflictions that combine with Apnea to ravage a body.** There is a steady progression of the incidence of Apnea in a population, followed by a decline among those of advanced age (a surprising factoid). The first critical point of the graph is to note the danger zone in the middle years. But the graph also highlights another important aspect of age and Apnea.

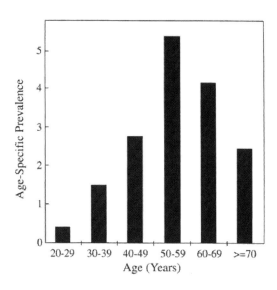

Apneacs who use maintenance treatments to keep their OSA at bay often make an assumption that may get them into trouble: the disease is NOT static.

Too many Apneacs believe that a sleep study from five or even ten years ago still reflects the reality of their disease. But old studies are not current. **The progression of Apnea is not static**. Things, especially our bodies, change over time. If an Apneac doesn't proactively keep up to-date with their TOOLs, like using the latest CPAP machines to maintain themselves against the onslaught of the disease, aging by itself can make Apnea worse. This is why this third predictor – age – should be heeded. Keep up to date. You will likely want to change your TOOLs to deal with a changing reality.

# PREDICTOR FOUR:

## Snoring Frequency

One measure of snoring is its prevalence in humor. It is real funny! In fact it's a staple of comedy. But snore humor enforces a systemic social tendency to deny that snoring is a real problem. Society is dismissive of snoring and almost portrays it as cute. Keep your guard up. It's another danger sign on your road of life.

To laugh at and ignore a danger sign is a disservice. Swimming in denial can leave you gasping for breath. Some may respond, "If only the sign was bigger." But frequent snoring is a BIG sign. Don't let the laughter blind you. **In any group of snorers, a large percentage of them will be Apneacs**. Many people snore; 30% to 50% of the US population snores at one time or another, some dangerously. On the other hand, snoring is not necessarily Apnea. It's important to distinguish between snoring and OSA. If you snore frequently, or snore loudly, which is predictor six, do yourself a favor: get diagnosed to determine whether (or not) you have Apnea.

## *What is Snoring?*

The noise of snoring is caused by parts of the nose and throat – generally referred to as the soft palate – vibrating with the in-and-out breath. During sleep, the soft palate is likely to become floppy and vibrate because the muscles of the airways have relaxed, causing then to narrow and vibrate, making a snore far more likely.

# Bernoulli

Really, really loud snoring can be explained by the work of a famous Dutch-Swiss mathematician, Daniel Bernoulli, born in 1700. He's particularly remembered for his applications of mathematics to fluid mechanics, or how fluid flows. Technically, both air and water are considered fluids, with air described as a compressible fluid. Bernoulli formulated an equation that describes how air flows and that, as it flows faster, a very non-intuitive thing happens. In short, for the purposes of snoring and Apnea, his work shows that when the airway passage becomes smaller and smaller due to obstruction or irritation, the pressure in that airway goes down, not up! And when air is forced to flow even faster through a very small soft opening, the pressure can actually reach zero. When this happens, the airway tissue is weirdly pulled together and not pushed apart. It's as if a magnet pulls the sides together, resulting in a loud vibration and an often-total obstruction of the small opening, until the air stops flowing.

# PREDICTOR FIVE:

## Waist Circumference

It's popular culture, we all know it; you can't avoid it, and it's literally right before your eyes: an increased waist circumference, or belt size, is one of several ways in which obesity affects the appearance of the body. And yet we try to deny it. Maybe we're just trying to be polite. Here's the fact: **a large waist is one of the most likely predictors or indicators of the dread worsening disease, Apnea**. Also discussed in Chapter 4 in the section on obesity, waist circumference depends a lot on omentum, one of the three kinds of fat in the human body.

The omentum is belly fat that hangs underneath the stomach muscles. Considered an organ, omentum fat is closest to the major organs and quickly accessible to the liver. We mention it again here because it complicates the simple observation, above, that waist circumference predicts Apnea. We'll address those complications in a subsequent chapter, Chapter 8, when we look into what is known about dieting effectively to Avenge Apnea.

# PREDICTOR SIX:

## Snoring Loudness

The final predictor of Apnea is how loud a person snores. **The louder you snore, the greater the chances that you will develop Apnea**. That is, if, in fact, you aren't already an

Apneac. It seems like there's not much more to say other than louder is worse and more often is worse, too. But what do we mean by loud? Or how bad can it get? How often? What about snoring so badly that no one, not even the snorer, can sleep? Again, Bernoulli's equation is useful here. Loud snoring is a result of massive airflow via a small or constricted airway. If the pressure in the airway goes to zero, cessation of airflow can result. So super loud snoring is at the dangerous end of the snoring continuum, very close to the next step, full-on obstruction. Hypopnea can also be a result of snoring and this means very little airflow occurs.

Workplace safety rules factor both the loudness of the sound, and the duration, or the amount of time you are exposed to that sound. Sound over 80-85 decibels is considered hazardous to hearing if exposure to the noise continues for long periods of time. And the more often it happens, the worse the impact on hearing.

## How Bad Can Snoring Get?

How bad can loud snoring get? Real bad. In fact, the world's loudest snorer, Mrs. Jenny Chapman of the UK was recorded at a whopping 111.6 decibels. Not quite a jackhammer, but close enough to ruin sleep for those in the area. As shown in the table below, Common Noises Expressed in Decibels, loud snoring averages at an eardrum-rattling 80 db.

| Common Noises Expressed in Decibels | Db |
| --- | --- |
| Whisper, rustling leaves | 30 |
| Average home noise | 40 |
| Conversational voice | 60 |
| Average snore | 62 |

| | |
|---|---|
| Alarm clock | 65 |
| Vacuum cleaner | 75 |
| Toilet flush | 75 |
| LOUD SNORE | 80 |
| Telephone ring | 80 |
| Pneumatic drill | 85 |
| Lawnmower | 87 |
| Chain saw | 90 |
| Shouted conversation | 90 |
| Motorcycle | 92 |
| Crying baby | 108 |
| Car horn | 110 |
| LOUDEST RECORDED SNORE | 112 |
| Subway train | 115 |
| Jet plane takeoff | 120 |
| Ambulance siren | 120 |
| Rock concert | 126 |
| Jackhammer | 130 |
| Balloon pop | 157 |
| Shotgun | 170 |

# Stealth Predictor:

## Inherited Traits

Another way to look at prediction is to look at inherited factors. This is a stealth factor, a predictor that may sneak up without having ever been noticed. It's literally Apnea in a person's genes. It's a factor that's interlaced with all six of the statistical predictors from the John's Hopkins – USC study.

Surprises come from all directions so it shouldn't be a surprise that OSA is inheritable. But it's a fact: relatives of those with OSA are themselves more likely to have Apnea. Chalk it up to family resemblance. It all boils down to this question: what is your airway inheritance? The relevant inheritable traits are complex, because in different combinations, they play out in various ways. Of two brothers with remarkable similarity who maintain similar health throughout their lives, one might have a slightly smaller chin, and be at greater risk for Apnea, while the other escapes the disease.

In a study evaluating 20 participants known to have Apnea and 40 of their as-yet-undiagnosed relatives, Apnea was found to be more prevalent among the relatives than within the general population. After undergoing a sleep study, 20% of the relatives were diagnosed with significant Apnea. By contrast, Apnea was diagnosed in only 5% of the random group. All 20 participants had a "normal" BMI, which further demonstrates that inheritable characteristics, not just weight, can be a predictor of Apnea.

## Apneac Profile

One of the great film directors of the 50's and 60's, Alfred Hitchcock's profile is perhaps one of the most famous of those time. He had a small chin, and large neck. And he was quite portly. He died in 1980 of renal failure, which is basically kidney disease. His oral cranial structure certainly causes one to think he may have been at risk for Apnea. As we know, Apnea can drive diabetes. And chronic renal failure is commonly driven by diabetes. Absent a late-breaking tell-all biography by one consort or another, we may never know for sure if he was an Apneac, but he was practically type-cast for Apnea.

Just like family resemblance (remarked most often about facial characteristics), physical traits like your craniofacial complex are inheritable. This is not simple. Inherited traits can be assembled with slightly different variations, leading to unique results, both as regards your looks and your airway. Your craniofacial complex is the configuration of your head, including your face, skull and oral cavities. Everyone has a unique craniofacial complex and it can be one of the most important heritable determinants of Apnea.

# Finding the Right Doctor

We'll close this chapter with a true story that brings together a number of key points from these first five chapters.

## D's Story

After a near-fatal episode of night terror one New Year's Eve, a friend we will refer to as "D" was given an expedited referral to the Stanford sleep disorder clinic. Neither the referral nor the night terrors were new to him, for in the previous decade he had endured multiple sleep studies, met nearly a dozen doctors, and been prescribed nearly every medication imaginable in a failed attempt to remedy the terrors. Nothing had worked.

From the start, the Stanford Clinic was different. A French neurologist, "a world renowned sleep specialist," examined him. Entering the exam room with his colleague, the French Doctor commented, "This is a classic case: look at his facial structure, the distance between his nose and chin is disproportionately long in comparison to his nose and forehead. This jaw configuration sets his tongue too far back, encouraging the collapse of his airway during sleep."

Turning his attention to D's nose, and pointing, the French Doctor continued, "Now look at the profile of his nose. See how the tip is slightly elevated? I bet he has a deviated septum."

Despite decades of suffering and numerous drugs and doctors, the deviated septum had never been noticed, much less diagnosed. Yet these observations were soon confirmed with an examination and breathing tests. After several nights at the clinic for "Sleep Studies" it was confirmed that D had mild Apnea together with a more severe Sleep Hypopnea, or shallow breathing at night with intermittent short periods of no respiration.

The following night D was fitted with a CPAP machine to determine how much pressure was required to keep his airway open and his breathing regular. In consultation, the doctors explained to D that Apnea and Hypopnea had recently been proven to be the most prevalent trigger for night terrors and sleepwalking. They also explained how irregular breathing unnaturally disturbs a person's slow wave sleep, thereby triggering night terrors and other sleep disorders.

The doctors told D that night terrors and similar disorders often appear among patients with such mild cases of disordered breathing that they don't even meet the classic definition of Apnea or Hypopnea.

Solutions available to D included a CPAP machine, surgical correction of his deviated septum to improve nasal airflow, and a rather extreme option, Maxillo-mandibular Advancement (MMA) surgery to open airway. Happily, D started with CPAP and he hasn't had an episode of night terrors since.

# CHAPTER 6:
# Overcoming Apnea

## *A Jock Strap for The Tongue*

*OSA had been with me for over 10 years and I'd just moved to a new city, so I decided to establish a relationship with "the best Apnea doctor in town." My family doctor told me whom to see. Right about here, I need to tell you that I'd had an extensive Apnea surgery at Stanford University Hospital by the leading area surgeon five years prior. The layman's term for that surgery is "tongue advancement combined with extensive microwaving of the nasal passage and removal of the floppy uvula in the back of the mouth." It was very painful and it took a long, long time to recover. Following recovery, tests showed it "did not" cure my Apnea. My AHI index was about the same as before.*

*So, when I finally got a slot to speak with "the best sleep doctor in town," I was pumped. The first ten minutes of my allotted fifteen were intense, "What's the latest research show about treatments that work?" I asked. "What exercises can be done? What's the likelihood that diet can work?" I was on a roll. "Is there a combination that's shown to reverse Apnea?" My questions were pouring out. Finally, "the best sleep doctor in town" tapped my knee to stop me, as he turned to a laminated poster on the wall and said, "Let me show you a new surgical procedure that supports your tongue by threading a wire from your chin through the mass of your tongue and back to your chin." I followed his finger across the graphic and nearly choked on my tongue as he explained how, "we then use a special key to tighten and adjust the wire." We looked at each other. I asked him about my questions. Sitting back down on his examination stool, he rolled closer. He leveled with me, speaking very softly "I don't know anything about your questions. I'm a surgeon. I operate. This is what I do. Let me know if you want the tongue suspension surgery." I already knew that tongue jock strap was not going to happen. That was the day I doubled my efforts to learn why Apnea happens and what options, beyond surgery, exist.*

*~W.E.H.*

# TOOLs

In prior chapters we told you about the horrors of Apnea, and over 30 highly correlated afflictions. Big-Fat-Bummers. Killer Afflictions. We also explained the predictors for Apnea and how those predictors, or indicators, relate to the correlated afflictions.

In this chapter, **we're going to switch gears. We want to tell you about the reasons for hope**, the reason we wrote this book.

Now that you understand what you are up against, we are going to start telling you the many, many approaches that are available to you to treat, and possibly even heal, Apnea. And we will use the rest of this book to do all the telling that there is to tell, because there is a lot of reason to hope. We call these reasons for hope "TOOLs."

An Apnea Avenger's TOOL is a device, method, approach, activity or behavior that may be useful to affect the severity and trajectory of the disease. In the same way that a wrench won't fit all bolts, these TOOLs are simply not going to work for all Apneacs in the same way, if at all. Some TOOLs work only when actively and routinely used. Other TOOLs prepare the body to continue a winning outcome long after the TOOL is employed.

But what is a TOOL? To say that we know how to apply a TOOL means that we have learned how to make something behave in a certain way (usually in a way that we prefer). If I'm controlling the car, I exercise my preference to make it go left or right by turning the steering wheel in the preferred direction.

Other devices, like a computerized word-processing program, have multiple TOOLs, nested in drop-down menus logically arranged according to task. These are like the drawers of a mechanic's toolbox. On the computer the menus differ according to tasks – as, for example, Printing or Editing. Similarly the mechanic's toolbox (of an organized mechanic, at least) has a drawer for screwdrivers, another for wrenches, and another for ratchets. You get the idea.

## Hi-Ho Silver!

Out on the Internet, for every malady that afflicts humanity there are one-shot solutions and promises of cures. It's no different with Apnea. While some may help or even work to ease or treat Apnea, it's just not that simple. **There is no silver bullet.**

**Apnea is a serious and complicated disease.** There are multiple inherited traits that may factor into the disease, and these are usually combined with a range of previous "self-inflicted lifestyle choices" to make each person's Apnea a unique, individual and often difficult challenge.

But there is good news. As we explained in Chapter 1, there are TOOLs. Rather, there is a TOOLbox, and there are three drawers in the Apneac's TOOLbox, with multiple TOOLs in each of the drawers. We will describe these drawers and their contents in greater detail further on in this chapter.

But right now, to give you a good glimpse of the organization that will be applied to the next half of the book, we don't think it's going to be overly repetitious to emphasize the overarching principle of the book. That said, the drawers are labeled: External, System and Targeted:

- ✓ **External TOOLs**
- ✓ **System TOOLs**
- ✓ **Targeted TOOLs**

Some of these TOOLs are quite simple and can be used – immediately – to both treat and curtail the advance of Apnea.

Sure, you may need to sleep with a device for the rest of your life, but if that's the TOOL that keeps you from falling into worse health, you're likely to find that it beats the alternative of a long decline towards an early death. That would be a maintenance TOOL. It enables you to stop the progression of Apnea and maintain your health, possibly improve it.

Abating, reversing or, ultimately, healing Apnea can be a bit trickier. Why? Because these variables: (1) the array of potential inherited traits, and (2) the range of lifestyle choices, and (3) the complicated feedback-loop interrelationship of inherited traits with lifestyle choices, make the prospect of healing or reversing OSA rather, shall we say, daunting. We're going to need something more adjustable and nimble than "ye old silver bullet." So we're going to show you some TOOLs that can be applied to specific areas of the body, and other TOOLs to treat your entire body – that's each and every one of your billions of cells.

## What is a "TOOL?"

At the risk of belaboring the point, we repeat: when we talk about a TOOL for the treatment of Apnea, it's an approach to improving the Apneac's condition. That can mean a number of things, ranging from abating, improving, or reversing and possibly even a complete healing.

Or, it may just mean effectively treating the symptoms of Apnea, at which prospect some might foolishly scoff as though "merely" maintaining the Apneac's health isn't enough.

## Mere Maintenance!

Stop. Merely? Maintaining an Apneac's health is a huge accomplishment, which both extends life and enhances life quality. **Do not underestimate the value of maintenance**. Maintenance is the baseline from which every Apnea Avenger must start their path to healing.

For although Apnea still remains a problem, maintenance is the key to preventing Apnea from progressing or triggering the unfortunate arrival of any one of the many unsavory characters, those dread afflictions that tag along with Apnea, bringing misery and worse.

## CPAP Defined

CPAP is a medical device, a breathing appliance that is worn at night. CPAP is the foremost TOOL available to reliably maintain the Apneac's health. **In nearly all cases, CPAP halts both the effects and the progression of OSA.** Further on in this chapter, we will delve into CPAP more fully. One crucial point that we cannot overemphasize: without CPAP, the lives of nearly all touched by Apnea would be miserable and hopeless.

# It's About Choices

We believe that the best option is to lay all the TOOLs out on the table and let each reader decide what his or her approach will be.

- ✓ Do you only want to halt the progression of Apnea, content to retain your current weight?

- ✓ Do you want to slim your neck and strengthen your airway?

- ✓ Do you want to do everything within your power to heal yourself?

It is your choice. Your choice may change over time. There is no right answer, but there is an answer that might be right for you.

Beginning with this, the first of the TOOLs chapters, we will use the remainder of this book to inform you of medically deployable approaches, effective devices and implements, and promising – even controversial – TOOLs.

We will also tell you what is presently known about other TOOLs, including proactive approaches that you can pursue: TOOLs that include specific exercises, diet and nutrition.

## Don't Obsess

No one Apneac can be expected to quickly and fully implement all TOOLs. That would be whiz-kid self-doctoring. It makes perfect sense to start by implementing one, or two, or a few TOOLs to some degree or other, perhaps with the intention that, over time, your first success will lead you to combine more TOOLs to better manage your Apnea, thereby reducing the likelihood that it will progress. Then, combined with growing self-awareness, understanding, and continuous personalized and knowledgeable application, overcoming and reversal can happen.

# Prior to CPAP, Romeo Routinely Died

Until 1981 when Dr. Sullivan developed the first CPAP machine, an open tracheotomy was the likely alternative to a slow death from Apnea. But this surgery was at best a problematic solution, prone to infection, needing to be plugged during the day. "Nice scarf, Romeo!" Besides the inconvenience, it formed an unsightly permanent throat wound, making an Apneac bed partner far less romantic even than a lunatic snorer. Before CPAP, Prince Apneac Romeo never had a chance.

## Not Negotiable

Every Apneac needs to establish a maintenance baseline with CPAP. But you might prefer to weigh less and so you could (literally) "exercise" your preference to weigh less by turning away from fattening and unhealthy foods. Or you might turn towards exercise. You could, so to speak, make a TOOL of the "weight knobs" by turning down the big knob from more to less, and turning the "quality dial" away from empty calories and towards healthy nutritious food. But you really should seriously begin with CPAP. Just remember, absent a miracle, any healing is a process; it takes patience, practice and persistence. So start with a baseline. Maintain your current health while you learn to address the disease from other angles. Start CPAP. Most super heroes have an ally. To be a successful Apnea Avenger, CPAP is your best choice.

## The Right TOOL for The Right Job

The next focus is on TOOLs that are known to work for Apneacs and are accessible to nearly everyone. Each of these basic TOOLs is designed to do the job, to help lower and then maintain lower AHI scores. AHI is the ultimate measureable result. Applied to your experience, AHI will tell you whether or not these TOOLs work for YOU.

### What's Our Definition of Works?

When your leg is broken and you cannot walk on your broken leg, a crutch works. It is an improvement. Remember, improvement is relative to your predicament.

Can't sleep? A CPAP machine that finally gets you a night of rest is an improvement. Can't enjoy romance with a CPAP tube on your face? Then try exercise or diet to reduce your Neck Circumference, finally allowing you to breathe; well, that, too, would be an improvement built upon the prior improvement, CPAP. Each improvement is likely to be unique, even incomparable.

For example, alone in the woods with a broken leg, lacking a crutch, a sturdy length of fallen tree limb works well; it is a tool to find control in a near-death predicament. Days later provided with crutches, that same stick is little more than a souvenir.

When things are broken, what works can be subjective but also both contextual and relative. Yes that is a slippery definition. But on a scale of 1-10, a reduction of pain, say, from an almost intolerable eight down to a bearable six ... well, wouldn't that probably be worthwhile?

# What's Working?

As more than one master craftsman has said, "It's never the tool, it's always how you work the tool that makes the work *work*."

## Apnea Avenger's TOOLbox

The Apneac Avenger's TOOLbox has three drawers, or menus (if you are a Geek) contained with in it. These are the External TOOLs, System TOOLs and Targeted TOOLs.

### External TOOLs

The term external indicates that these TOOLs are applied to the body either every night, such as CPAP or a dental mouth guard appliance, or perhaps represent a one-time application like a surgical implantation of Dacron strings in the soft throat tissue to provide lasting stiffening of the flabby tissues implicated in OSA. (We do not consider an irreversible and invasive surgery, such as mandibular advancement, a TOOL. Such medical treatment is incompatible with the concept of TOOLs in this book.)

The benefits that External TOOLs bring to the entire system may be permanent (surgery) or transient (CPAP). While External TOOLs often have positive effects on OSA and other chronic afflictions, the benefits may be limited by other issues, such as the skill of the surgeon, or the proper adjustment of the CPAP. External TOOLs are just one of three drawers in the Apnea Avenger's TOOLbox, which also includes System TOOLs and Targeted TOOLs.

- ✓ CPAP is one of the External TOOLs.

- ✓ Reversible Surgeries are External TOOLs.

- ✓ Dental Appliances are also External TOOLs.

### System TOOLs

System TOOLs are strategies for healing that work on the entire body. They are global in their application and in their impact. The benefits that System TOOLs bring to the entire system have positive effects on OSA and many other chronic afflictions.

Examples of System TOOLs are Weight Loss and Global Exercise. For now, don't let this brief overview fool you: this is a big TOOL drawer.

- ✓ Weight Loss is one of the System TOOLs.

- ✓ Global Exercise is one of the System TOOLs.

### Targeted TOOLs

Targeted TOOLs work on specific parts or systems of the body. These are area-specific methods for obtaining specific results in specific parts of the body. They are focused on specific problems that are involved in the larger picture of Apnea. But don't let this specificity narrow your vision. The benefit of Targeted TOOLs is that the health of the entire system can be improved by addressing one specific area of the body. For example, there are sets of TOOLs that can be used to target Neck Circumference, which is directly implicated with Apnea and which – when strengthened, toned and slimmed – correlates directly with an improvement in the Apneac's condition. Such targeted improvements have positive effects on OSA and many of the other chronic afflictions that are highly correlated with Apnea.

- ✓ Circular Breathing is one of the Targeted TOOLs.

- ✓ Playing a musical wind instrument such as the Didgeridoo is one of the Targeted TOOLs.

- ✓ Oropharyngeal Exercise is one of the Targeted TOOLs.

- ✓ Isometric Gum-chewing (aka Gum Control) is one of the Targeted TOOLs.

- ✓ Targeted Yoga is one of the Targeted TOOLs.

## The End of Denial Is A Turn-On

Now the first TOOL, which really is the "on switch" of your health TOOLbox, is to make the big choice, now. You need to grab hold and take charge of your health. That will mark the end of denial. Take control of your health by taking charge of your healing. Get the TOOLs and get going. Of course, you can wait and decide later. It's your health. It's your life that's wasting.

# No Change Without Measurement

### Trust But Verify

You may trust yourself to know what has changed, but without regular consistent measurements, or a visit to your Aunt every year for Thanksgiving, you won't really know. **Nothing is definite without measurement**. While it might seem easier to endure some cheek pinching as Auntie exclaims, "Oh, my Harold, you've lost so much weight!" your nighttime breathing patterns can be measured and recorded. The biggest difference being that you get to be the turkey.

There are several measurement methods and scales for the assessment of Apnea and other sleep disorders. The tests and corresponding measurements differ mainly in what they are intended to measure, which explains the range of methods, which include a self-administered questionnaire, blood samples, and sophisticated computerized machines that hook the patient (turkey) up with cords, sensors and monitors. We favor the AHI (Apnea-Hypopnea Index) method because it is very measurable, less subjective and is repeatable.

## Measuring Apnea

According to ResMed, "partner-observed snoring with cessation of breathing" is the number one predictor of Apnea. But partner observation doesn't usually tell the Apneac much about their condition. "You kept me up all night for the third night in a row, HAROLD!" doesn't really tell him how severe his condition is, nor does it improve his disposition to hide behind a mountain of denial. Even if she were to have calmly shared that she's become concerned, and begun taking notes and finally then told him, "I'm concerned. It's not about my losing sleep, it's about me not losing you. Oh, Harold, dear, you stop breathing. Completely. And it happens at least four times, every hour, throughout the night. Sometimes it's worse. I'm concerned."

Even at that point, while the disease may be evident, the denial may likely be impenetrable. That's where a recording device or the medical sleep clinic becomes so valuable. One reason is that it becomes harder to resist data than it is to deny charts compiled by bedmates. Another is that, even with an accurate measurement of breaths per hour, the diagnosis of Apnea is not entirely complete.

Greater accuracy can be obtained regarding the kind and severity of the Apnea. That's because there are other factors that can be measured with sleep instrumentation. For example, Hypoxia (when breathing is happening but not enough air is coming through to keep the blood oxygen saturation at normal levels) is not easily counted. And the AHI is a combination of the two – cessation of breathing and low airflow.

Luckily, the gamut of modern sleep instrumentation begins with the simple but practical finger clip and extends off to the realm of complicated measurements and sleep laboratories. And when it comes to continued measurement, maintenance and treatment of the disease, there are both consumer-level sleep devices such as the Lark, and physician-prescribed Apnea machines, or Continuous Positive Airway Pressure (CPAP) machines.

## Sleep Centers or Labs

Sleep centers or labs are medical facilities that are outfitted with monitoring equipment designed to diagnose sleeping disorders. **Patients spend the night at a sleep lab, where they sleep painlessly connected to monitors that accurately detect and distinguish between OSA, CSA, Mixed Apnea**, or even variants such as positional OSA, and then develop a response with CPAP. All often accomplished in one night.

## Apnea-Hypopnea Index

The most common way to measure the severity of Apnea is the Apnea-Hypopnea Index, or AHI. It's intuitively easy to understand, since it measures how many times a person wakes in one hour. It is not subjective, so it's considered an accurate measure of Apnea, and is used almost universally to rate the severity the disease. It is used to describe the severity of both complete Apnea and partial obstruction as with Hypopnea. **Mild Apnea** is in the range of 5-15 interruptions per hour; **Moderate Apnea**, 15-30; and **Severe Apnea** occurs with more than 30 interruptions of sleep per hour.

As shown in the following table, AHI scales the severity of Apnea – ranging from Mild, to Moderate, to Severe – based on the total number of breathing cessations lasting more than 10 seconds, per one hour of sleep.

| Apnea Severity | Interruptions / Hour |
|---|---|
| Mild | 5-15 |
| Moderate | 15-30 |
| Severe | 30 or more |

The Apnea-Hypopnea Index (AHI) is measured by a device that is available either through an overnight visit to a sleep lab, or in-home with a special "sleep device."

# Partner Observed Measurement

Obviously, if you are the Apneac, you cannot count the number of times your sleep is disturbed in an hour, but the partner whom you are keeping awake probably can. Finally an Apneac agrees to be tested. Once you know how many times an Apneac wakes per hour, it's simple math to calculate the AHI: just take the total number of Apnea events, or episodes, plus the total number of Hypopnea events, divided by that number by the total number of sleep-time minutes, and multiply that result by 60 (minutes).

## Elephants in the Overnight Sleep Study Room

Many Apneacs, convinced they're "probably not that bad," are surprised to find they have a high AHI index. That's the elephant in the overnight sleep study room: the higher the number, the bigger the elephant. A high AHI index tells the Apneac how often they wake in their sleep and just how far they must climb to get over their denial.

## Desaturation Measurement (or, Oxygen Saturation)

This test is the bottom line. It measures what any person with a breathing problem needs to know: **Is there enough oxygen in your blood to support healthy body functions?**

**Oxygen is critical for life.** In medicine, oxygen saturation refers to oxygenation of the blood. Our blood is pumped by the heart throughout the circulation system of veins and arteries. When it reaches the lungs, it is "oxygenated." Oxygenation occurs when the lungs take oxygen molecules from that air and transfers them to the blood. From there, the blood continues circulation and distributes the oxygen to the tissues of the body.

One advantage of a Desaturation Measurement is that the Oxygen saturation measurements can be obtained with a clip on the end of the index finger. The measurement is obtained using a near-infrared spectroscopy (NIRS) sensor. This differs substantially from testing for AHI, which requires an overnight stay for evaluation in a sleep lab with multiple electrodes connected to all parts of the body.

Desaturation Measurement determines the amount of the oxygen in the blood, which will be lower with OSA/Apnea events, caused by the act of not breathing or such shallow breathing that it leads to Hypoxia. Technically, it is a measure of the percentage of hemoglobin binding sites in the bloodstream that are occupied by oxygen. The scale for Desaturation Measurement is quite narrow.

**A Desaturation Measurement of 95% is considered normal. But a measurement of 88% or below often qualifies someone for supplemental oxygen.** Even though it's the bottom line, this test can't pinpoint the cause. Obviously, it is important to know what is driving the low blood saturation. So, taken alone, Desaturation Measurement just tells how big the problem is, but requires further testing to determine how to treat it.

## The Multiple Sleep Latency Test (MSLT)

The main purpose of the MSLT, or Multiple Sleep Latency Test is to obtain an objective measure of sleepiness. With the MSLT, sleepiness is measured by the time it takes to fall asleep. The diagnostic tool measures the time elapsed from the start of daytime nap period to the first signs of sleep. The elapsed time is called sleep latency.

**The MSLT can be used to distinguish between physical tiredness and true excessive daytime sleepiness**. It's also used to assess whether treatments for breathing disorders are working.

## Epworth Sleepiness Scale

Also used to measure and diagnose sleep disorders, the Epworth Sleepiness Scale measures a person's perception of how tired and sleepy they feel. Called, "daytime sleepiness," **the Epworth scale provides a diagnostically relevant score based on the answers to eight self-administered questions**. Introduced in 1991 by Dr. Murray Johns in Australia, the Epworth Sleepiness Scale is a subjective tool offering a different perspective of an Apneac's situation. For example, if the cause of sleepiness is not being caused by cessation of breathing, someone might score high on the Epworth and not on the AHI. Although it is clearly a subjective measurement, the Epworth Sleepiness Scale remains an important diagnostic tool.

## Calgary Sleep Apnea Quality of Life Index (SAQLI)

Apnea has been shown to adversely affect patients' quality of life. Although the physiologic measures, such as the Epworth, and symptom scales, such as the AHI, may fail to adequately measure the true impact of the disorder on each person, a measurement like **the Calgary Sleep Apnea Quality of Life Index (SAQLI) helps patients to recognize and compare how they feel before CPAP treatment begins and then after it has been administered**. This simple measurement is often used in hospital settings. The Calgary Sleep Apnea Quality of Life Index (SAQLI) is a disease-specific quality of life questionnaire developed to measure how an Apneac's life changes in response to a therapeutic intervention. It is essentially a before-and-after evaluation of therapies.

## Measure for Measure

As you will learn in the following chapters of this book, the core of the "Sleep or Die" method for the treatment, reversal and possible healing of Apnea is to;

- ✓ Measure.
- ✓ Use a TOOL.
- ✓ Measure Again.
- ✓ Based on the Findings of the Measurement, Adjust Treatment and TOOLs.
- ✓ Use More TOOLs.
- ✓ Mind Your Attitude and Maintain Your Commitment.
- ✓ Repeat.

It's like learning to run a mile. You run. You measure your time on the first try. Then you train, measure, run the mile again. You compare the first time with the second. To ensure that you are training effectively, you might occasionally use a device like a heart monitor to help know just how you well your sprints and longer runs are preparing you for "the mile." Then you measure that next run. You adjust your training by adding or subtracting TOOLs (more or less sprints, more or less distance training). Repeat.

# TOOL Sets

Earlier in this chapter, we introduced the TOOLbox that's available for the Apneac to work with their disease. We have identified three sets, or drawers of TOOLs that are in the Apneac's TOOLbox. These are External TOOLs, System TOOLs, and Targeted TOOLs.

The **External TOOLs** are more-or-less passive methods applied to the body to either arrest or abate the symptoms. In the case of surgery, that's an attempt to cut the problem away, but without really addressing the potentially deeper causes; hence, the somewhat less than 100% satisfaction.

**System TOOLs** and **Targeted TOOLs** are more proactive approaches. **System TOOLs** are strategies for healing that are applied to the entire body, such as diet and exercise. **Targeted TOOLs** are practices for obtaining results in specific areas of the body; they are aimed at areas of the body that are involved in Apnea, such as the tongue, neck and throat.

# External TOOLs

## CPAP

This TOOL ensures reliable consistent nighttime breathing. Development of the Continuous Positive Airway Pressure (CPAP) machine in the early 1980's was the first step towards treatment of Apnea in what we would regard a positive, healthy, therapeutic manner.

**Prior to CPAP, a ghastly permanent tracheotomy was the Apneac's first, last and only option.** CPAP cleverly pushes air into the airway with a bit of pressure. That positive air pressure inflates the airway and creates more breathing room to prevent collapse and occlusion. It literally pushes the offending tissue out of the way with pressure.

## Surgeries

Since OSA is an oral-cranial problem involving inherited traits combined with excess neck fat, or what can be called a plumbing issue, perhaps changing the plumbing makes sense. OSA surgeries do just that. By moving a large tongue forward via surgery, the air "pipe" or airway has more room for air. By removing large tonsils, more room is made. By reducing the size of an overly large nasal turbinate, a bigger passage or "pipe" is created.

But these surgeries are usually irreversible, permanent, and sometimes involve complications that can worsen rather than improve the quality of the Apneac's life. Surgery makes better sense when other options have been exhausted.

## Appliances

Wearing a dental mouthpiece, which are commonly called "dental appliances" may make more breathing room. These options are a well-trodden path and success varies based on both the appliance and what's reducing the breathing room or collapsing the "pipes." These are a reversible, non-permanent option that may bring immediate relief.

# System TOOLs

## Diet & Weight Loss Through Diet

Achieving and maintaining a healthy weight addresses the heavy issue of " being overweight". While not exactly the same thing, weight loss and diet are inevitably connected, like opposite sides of the same coin. In researching the dots that connect known, published precursors to Apnea and likely companion diseases we found that, after CPAP, **weight loss ranks second for easing, managing, and possibly even healing Obstructive Sleep Apnea**. Weight loss, that is, through a conscious healthy diet. Weight loss creates more breathing room by reducing or ridding the neck area of heavy fat that works in conjunction with gravity to obstruct breathing. For the vast majority of Apneacs, this is the most effective TOOL. Why? **The vast majority of Apneacs are considered medically "overweight or obese."** For this population, being overweight may not be the only thing going on, but it's a big contributor.

An appropriately heavy chapter in this book, Chapter 8, is dedicated to new information about weight loss. Forget what you ate to get into this fix; learn how to eat your way out of it with Chapter 8 and lose weight.

## Global, or Full Body Exercise

Exercise is a healthy part of any balanced program to ease, manage and possibly even heal Apnea. Our emphasis is on exercise that most benefits the Apneac, which includes general exercise leading to overall weight loss, as well as proven specific exercises that target the number-one predictor of Apnea: Neck Circumference.

# Targeted or Specialized TOOLs

## Circular Breathing

Other ways to make more breathing room in the airway is to make it stronger, thus reinforcing the existing pipes and toning floppy tissues like the tongue. This TOOL, derived from the musical world of wind instruments, is explained in Chapter 9.

## Oral-Cranial-Facial Exercise

"Use it or lose it" resonates with everyone. Comedian Jerry Seinfeld was once asked why he continues to do stand-up comedy even though he is retired from his hit show and very wealthy. He quipped – "use it or lose it." For multitudes of reasons, our neck, tongue, cheeks, and airway become weak and flaccid. Targeted-exercise of these muscles makes them stiffer and stronger, resulting in less collapse and more breathing room at night.

# Apply Yourself

In the next chapter we're going to delve into the details of External TOOLs, which are described above as "more-or-less passive methods applied to the body to either arrest or abate the symptoms." But please don't think that you can have a passive approach to Apnea. **Apnea is aggressive. It will kill you**. We want you to be aggressive in your response; we want you to become an Apnea Avenger. Apnea Avengers will wisely make use of the appropriate External TOOLs to support them as they advance in their exploration of the other two drawers in the Apneac's TOOLbox.

Apnea Avengers, read on!

# CHAPTER 7:
# Get It On Just to Sleep

## The Solution is to Cut Your Legs Off...

*Carpenters swing hammers, cooks cook, surgeons cut. If you consult a carpenter about a problem, their view of the problem often looks like a nail in need of a good pounding. So it goes. Several years ago, a good friend injured his knee. A real athlete, he was fun to ski with, dominated the basketball games at the gym, and loved to be active. But that knee injury sidelined him – although he did manage to keep walking, "Just to stay fit." He consulted all kinds of experts without much luck. Then one day a mutual friend informed him that he was, "Totally in luck." A renowned knee surgeon from back east was coming to a conference in town, and had graciously agreed to see our friend about his knee. Thrilled, my friend met up with the "rock star" of knees in the lobby where the conference was held. With a quick lookover, the doctor gave him the answer. "You have an alignment issue, so we will just cut off both of your legs at the shin bone, move them to the right an inch or so and reattach them. This will solve your problem." Depressed, my friend left and limped several miles back home. On the way he happened by his chiropractor's office and thought, "My back is so tight, I think I'll stop in for an adjustment." So he did. Then he*

*continued the walk home – but something was different;*
*his knee did not hurt. Not just for that afternoon, but*
*evermore (with only an occasional back adjustment).*

*~W.E.H.*

# Three External TOOLs

As introduced in the previous chapter, the Apnea Avenger's TOOLbox contains three drawers holding the External TOOLs, System TOOLs and Targeted Exercise TOOLs.

Here, we will talk in depth about the three sets of TOOLs in the External TOOLs drawer. These are CPAP, Reversible Surgeries, and Dental Appliances.

External TOOLs are essentially *applied* to the body every night, such as CPAP or a dental mouth guard appliance, or may perhaps represent a one- time yet reversible invasion as with the surgical implantation of Dacron strings in the soft throat tissue to provide lasting stiffening of flabby tissue implicated in OSA. Accordingly, the benefits that External TOOLs bring to the entire bodily system may be permanent (surgeries) or transient (CPAP, etc.).

External TOOLs can also be something that you wear (Dental Appliances) only to spit out in the morning. While they often have positive effects on OSA and other chronic afflictions, the benefits of External TOOLs may be limited by other issues, such as the skill of the surgeon, or the proper adjustment of the CPAP. External TOOLs are just one of three drawers in the Apnea Avenger's TOOLbox, which also includes System TOOLs and Targeted TOOLs.

✓ CPAP and Other Breathing Devices are External TOOLs.

✓ Reversible Surgeries are External TOOLs.

✓ Dental Appliances are also External TOOLs.

Note: In order to be thorough, we include several of the more prevalent surgeries in this chapter. We do not consider irreversible invasive surgery, such as mandibular advancement, a TOOL. Surgeries of this order are incompatible with the concept of TOOLs in this book.

# CPAP

CPAP is a non-invasive means of treating Obstructive Sleep Apnea, or OSA. The Apneac sleeps with a mask or nasal interface connected by a flexible air tube to a small, specialized portable medical air compressor, or pump, that supplies room air at a positive pressure through the mask or nasal interface. The Apneac patient breathes in from the flow generator and exhales through a port in the mask. This creates continuous air pressure that, applied in this manner, acts as a pneumatic splint to keep the upper airway open and unobstructed.

An unfortunate 1% of Apneacs suffer from CSA. CSA involves an intermittent failure of the brain to send breathing signals; this is a complication in addition to the presence of OSA. CSA machines are more expensive and must be sized and tuned for the individual. That's because these machines provide both positive and negative air pressure whenever the brain forgets to breathe, essentially acting as a stand-by resuscitator throughout the night.

## The Argument for CPAP

CPAP is effective in halting the advance of OSA, while treating the symptoms of the disease. Logically, we can expect that the Apneac who stops using CPAP will be poorly rested and experience tiredness during the day. But what's much worse is that **when Apneacs go off treatment they become susceptible to all of the highly correlated diseases and afflictions – also known as Big-Fat-Bummers and Killer Afflictions –** detailed in Chapters 3 and 4. What's nice about CPAP is, once applied, some of the correlated afflictions improve – like ED, where 75% of the participants saw an immediate reversal, or uptick in function.

### CSA? or CSA CPAP (BiPAP)? or Mixed CPAP (VPAP Adapt SV)?

CPAP has become an imprecise umbrella term frequently applied to describe any ventilator used for the treatment of OSA, CSA or Mixed Apnea. But these different forms of Apnea each require specialized breathing devices.

# Terminological Confusion

Although Obstructive Sleep Apnea is often referred to as OSA, in the literature it is often shortened to Apnea. Central Sleep Apnea is spelled out completely or else shortened to CSA. We find that Mixed Sleep Apnea is referred to as Mixed, Mixed Apnea, or Mixed Events; yet the acronym MSA is not in common use. According to context, Apnea may refer to all three variants of sleep disturbed breathing, or just OSA. In this book, we attempted to abide by the observed inconsistent conventions of the Apnea literature, with occasional redundancies to make things clear.

## CSA CPAP (BiPAP)

Central Sleep Apnea (CSA) involves a brain misfire whereby the sleeper forgets to breathe. The complications of Central Sleep Apnea require a special, more finely tuned BiPAP machine to auto-breathe a sleeper through a CSA event. BiPap requires high and low pressure settings to successfully auto-breathe during a CSA event.

## Mixed CPAP (VPAP Adapt SV)

Neither CPAP nor BiPAP therapy alleviates the sleep disorders of Mixed Apnea (MSA) sufferers. In fact, treatment with CPAP or BiPAP can leave them with an elevated AHI, and the Apnea is not treated. Luckily for these Apneacs, research has led to another level of CPAP; like ResMed's VPAP Adapt SV, which uses adaptive servo-ventilation to adapt to a patient's ventilatory needs on a breath-by-breath basis.

## CPAP WORKS

**Any treatment that halts the advance of a degenerative disease can be said to "work." CPAP works**. Also, because we know that Apnea is a precursor of other afflictions, implementation of a CPAP therapy helps to prevent Apnea from triggering such correlated afflictions as stroke, heart disease and diabetes. **But a treatment program is a maintenance therapy, not a healing**. Think of CPAP as external support while you build up your internal support. Like scaffolding holding up the building walls while rebuilding the frame internally. As long as the scaffolding is in place, the building won't get worse or collapse. But scaffolding alone can't keep the building standing. CPAP is like that. It is a godsend for

Apneacs and their family and neighbors; in fact we all owe a heartfelt thanks to Peter Farrell and Dr. Colin Sullivan, early pioneers of the first CPAP machines.

So CPAP is not a cure. The industry acknowledges this. ResMed, a company which designs and develops CPAP machines on the original efforts of Sullivan and Farrell, states in their annual disclosures that CPAP is a treatment and not a cure and that it must be worn nightly. Still, in order for Apnea suffers to ease or reverse the severity of their disease, **CPAP provides the necessary stability in order for the healing process to begin**. Furthermore, without CPAP, companion ailments can make it very difficult, if not impossible, to recover. Sadly, with the undiagnosed rate of Apnea in the US hovering above 80%, most Apneacs will never see the benefits of CPAP. The bottom line is that CPAP works to maintain an Apneac's health and prevent the disease from progressing. It's far preferable to a tracheotomy, which is when an air hole is cut in one's throat below just the Adam's apple in order to allow a person to continue breathing when the normal throat airway is blocked by an Apnea event.

## CPAP Maintenance

For patients successfully treating their condition with a CPAP machine, **we cannot over-emphasize the importance of regular, if not monthly, adjustment to the device and its attachments, like facemasks**. Modern CPAP machines have microprocessors and features like removable SD cards, which are memory cards similar to those used in cameras. These cards are used to record breathing activity, mask leakage and other breath-relevant data.

> Doctors should review these results on a regular basis to make adjustments to ensure proper pressure and airflow; otherwise, patients may not receive the benefit of the machine. This can be one reason why other highly correlated afflictions appear to resume or even worsen after using CPAP for some time.

The clear benefits of CPAP aside, the focus of this book is for those who wish to overcome AND reverse the condition, when possible. This book may also provide solutions for those who can't or will not tolerate CPAP due to physical, emotional, or financial circumstances. However **it's interesting and thought provoking to note that, once fitted with CPAP, the most frequent question our sleep lab contact is asked is, "What exercises should I do?"** People want to heal, not survive one night at a time, strapped to a machine. While that's probably due to a long list of personal reasons, including self-image and the perception that CPAP presents an impediment, it can be embarrassing. So, for those who want a healing, it's time to go to the next level. That's why we wrote this book.

## When CPAP Does Not Work

Not all Apneacs are successfully managed or treated with CPAP. Some cannot or simply-will-not tolerate going to bed wrapped in an apparatus. They might be claustrophobic, or too vain and egotistic to submit to the indignity of sleeping piped to a machine. Others, locked in denial, obtain the diagnosis and the equipment, but never use it because that would require the Apneac to overcome denial. For still others, the impracticality of frequent power outages, large batteries, or frequent travel to non-grid locations (including camping) may crimp a regular CPAP regimen.

# Knife

As stated previously, in order to be thorough, we include several of the more prevalent surgeries thought to improve life for Apneacs. However, we do not consider irreversible invasive surgery, such as mandibular advancement, a TOOL.

# Surgery, Reversible Surgeries

Before CPAP, the primary treatment for OSA was a tracheotomy, a surgical procedure to cut a hole in the patient's windpipe to create a channel for airflow. It works but it is medieval. One of the common surgical treatments is uvulopalatopharyngoplasty (UPPP), which is a surgery of the upper airway to remove excess tissue and streamline the shape of the airway. Another surgery is like a permanent punch to the inside of the jaw; this most extreme surgery is almost Orwellian in its common name: Mandibular Advancement. Since we're not pulling any punches in this book, we'll tackle the worst first.

### Mandibular Advancement

Of common surgical solutions for Apneacs, maxillomandibular advancement ranks among the highest. And lowest. The idea behind this surgery is that the upper and lower jaws restrict the Apneac's airway. It is thought that, by surgically moving the upper and lower jaw forward, the entire airway will be opened and enlarged and that the Apnea will disappear. Usually the tongue is repositioned in the process. Too often it's the patient's money and health that disappear, while the Apnea retains its evil grip on their breathing. Of course **moving the jaws requires that the mouth is basically taken apart and reassembled differently**. According to the surgeons,

"This procedure serves as the most effective surgical treatment for Obstructive Sleep Apnea. It is performed on patients with moderate to severe Obstructive Sleep Apnea as the only treatment, or when other procedures have failed." Performed in a hospital under general anesthesia, the surgery itself requires three to four hours, followed by several days in the hospital and a month of healing before returning to work. The surgeons note that, "some changes in facial appearance will occur but is usually quite acceptable." **With a less than 100% success rate, however, it can be difficult to accept your results if you fall within the unsuccessful group**. There should be no question where our sympathies lie in regards to this surgery.

## Goetz Gets It

One of the pivotal inputs in the early phases of this project was a TED talk by the editor of Wired Magazine, Thomas Goetz, on the bland topic, "It's Time to Redesign Medical Data." The talk can be found online at the TED site. (Go to: www.ted.com & search for Thomas Goetz.) In his talk, Goetz alerts us all to the importance of useable medical data in the context of our own individual diagnosis. As he proceeds to explain how too little medical data is in fact usable by the patient, he opens the question, "What can you do?" He then offers a series of questions that every patient should ask. These questions are:

✓ Can I have my results?

✓ What does this mean?

✓ What are my options?

✓ What next?

Far from encouraging patients to be obnoxious, Goetz champions that idea that we can change lives and save ourselves from disappointing outcomes by adopting new behavior, encouraging open engagement vs. blind compliance with the mechanized medical establishment.

## UPPP and Other Surgeries

Uvulopalatopharyngoplasty (UPPP) is a common surgical treatment for Apnea. This is surgery of the upper airway to remove excess tissue and streamline the shape of the airway. Implemented alone, **UPPP has a poor success rate**, as it only targets one of the six obstruction points in the airway. Surgeons claim a better success rate when this procedure is combined with multi-stage upper airway surgical procedures. All these combined procedures are expensive, require highly specialized surgeons and often involve prolonged, painful recovery periods.

Other surgeries may implant a device to permanently stiffen and add support to the soft palate or, as in extreme cases, completely remodel the patient's mouth and face. Sometimes, obstruction in the nasal passages or a deviated septum creates a blockage of the patient's airway, causing Apnea.

Surgical correction of these issues may resolve the Apnea, or not.

Nearly all Apnea surgeries are irreversible, while non-invasive actions, like exercise, have no such burden and are both accessible to all at relatively low cost, with or without insurance, and offer real measurable benefits. Furthermore, when it comes to correcting Apnea, surgical success stories are, at best, spotty.

# No Going Back

For example, Mandibular Advancement, the surgery used on Will to move the tongue forward and thereby "cure" Apnea had a 30% failure rate. Many people focus optimistically on the greater chance of success, as did Will. But many who have the procedure without success wind up no better, sometimes worse, and in any case, about $25,000 lighter.

But this is no way to lose weight. Even among those for whom the procedure is considered successful, there are frequent unfortunate side effects, such as numb teeth lasting even a decade later. Will met with one doctor who used to do the surgeries but after counting the unhappy patients who had not benefited and the really unhappy ones who litigated, he stopped the surgeries, remarking, "CPAP is a much easier solution."

## Reversible Surgeries

It is the nature of surgery that, until now, surgeries were irreversible. However, a new class of surgeries is emerging; these are surgeries that implant a medical device with minimal tissue damage.

### Jock Strap for The Tongue

This is a somewhat reversible surgical procedure that involves the placement of a Dacron string within the tongue, which is then attached to the front of the jaw and tightened to suspend the tongue and thereby prevent it from sliding back to block the throat. Kind of like a high-tech jock strap for the tongue.

### Pillar Method

The most well known new reversible Apnea procedure is referred to as the "Pillar Method." Developed by Medtronic, this is a procedure where small medical Dacron tubes are implanted in the soft tissues of the upper back of the palate. The goal is to stiffen the soft tissue and prevent collapse while sleeping. Think of it as providing inner scaffolding, like rebar, within the tissue.

Depending on the air passage issue contributing to each Apneac's OSA, this can be a successful control. Here's the best part: if it's not working, the doctor can pull the tubes out and "leave no trace behind." Medtronic stipulates that, ultimately, the degree of improvement depends on the Apneac to address other contributing factors contributing to the OSA, like obesity. But if the Apneac fails to do their share, results vary accordingly.

# Dental Appliances

## About Dental Appliances

Dental appliances work to relieve Apnea by pulling the tongue away from the upper airway just enough to let air flow. Although not effective in all cases, mild Apnea can usually be helped by wearing such an appliance at night. Dental appliances are also helpful to CPAP users. Many of the more comfortable masks blow air into the nose and do not cover the mouth. Some users like the comfort but have a problem with air leaking out of their mouths and waking up. **A dental appliance usually helps keep the mouth from opening enough to allow air to rush out**. Dental appliances can also lower the CPAP effort, and therefore increase the Apneac's comfort, by pulling the tongue away from the back of the throat.

Depending on a person's physiology, specifically the configuration (shape), dimensions, and fitness of the various parts of the airway, from nose to lungs, a dental appliance may be sufficient to provide relief from Apnea. But as with all things Apneac, it may be ineffective for others. For example, an Apneac with a large tongue and a large air passage may find that a dental appliance provides the best and simplest therapy, while it might be ineffective for another person with a smaller airway.

Since Apnea issues can arise from dysfunctions that may occur anywhere from the tip of the nose all the way down to the lungs, a person with a severely deviated septum and a small tongue might not be helped at all by dental appliances. Yet it's often the case that both CPAP and a dental appliance together will work better for some individuals than either one separately. Dental appliances work with the tongue, not the muscles of the airway, so although they may work in the right circumstances, they are not always effective. But they are not permanent, not terribly expensive, and are worth trying; certainly before any surgery is ever considered, or as an assistive crutch while the Apneac turns their attention to other TOOLs.

## Other TOOLs

System TOOLs, such as whole body exercise and diet, as well as Targeted TOOLS, which include specific exercises that focus on the throat and neck, are far more empowering to the person and more likely to lead to lasting results over a lifetime.

In the following chapter, we turn to Diet. For nearly all Apneacs, **Diet is likely the most powerful TOOL in the Apneac's TOOLbox.**

So put down your spoon and dig into it.

# CHAPTER 8:
# At A Loss For Sleep

## *The Right Diet Starts at The Start*

*I spoke with a well-known orthodontist and his fiancé who do humanitarian work and research among the Inuit above the Artic Circle. Talking about Apnea, he shared a theory pointing to the importance of breast-feeding in preventing OSA. An incredible puzzle piece may have been found, for it appears that breast-feeding may be a factor in predicting this disease, starting only moments after birth!*

*When a baby is given a diet of breast milk and it is delivered via the nipple, the sucking motion spreads out the mouth box because it is very pliable when young. This gives the teeth more room to spread out and the baby grows up with less dental issues. Plus, it creates a bigger area for the tongue! According to this orthodontist friend, the spike of OSA in the Inuit population correlates with the age group born when the tribes began to bottle-feed their newborn babies.*

*~WEH*

# Wait, There's More!

In the last chapter we introduced the first TOOL drawer in the Apnea Avenger's TOOLbox, the External TOOLs. We described the most passive approaches to treating and resolving the symptoms of Apnea.

But wait! There's much more! More to do, and more to lose. And that's the central point of this chapter.

Most Apneacs have weight to lose, and they should not wait to begin. That's largely because the modern diet of refined carbohydrates floods our blood with excess sugars, adversely affecting the metabolism, and respiratory muscles, eventually leading to weight gain and poor health.

If for no other reason, this chapter on weight loss could be the heaviest chapter of the book on healing Apnea. Ironically, in an earlier, simpler society – likely with a much simpler and healthier diet – there would be almost nothing to say. We will keep it light.

Apnea of course, usually involves poor health and excess weight. Diet revamping is an idea that fits, even if the pants don't. Diet is one very effective way to reverse the Apnea diagnosis while you drop a waist size or two; diets do improve breathing.

# Weight Loss TOOL: Diet

Weight Loss is one of the primary System TOOLs.

## System TOOLs

System TOOLs work on the entire body. The benefits that System TOOLs bring to the entire system have positive effects on OSA and other chronic afflictions. Examples of System TOOLs are

Weight Loss and Global Exercise. System TOOLs are just one of three drawers in the Apnea Avenger's TOOLbox, which also includes External TOOLs and Targeted TOOLs.

✓ Weight Loss is one of the System TOOLs.

✓ Global Exercise is one of the System TOOLs.

### Just A Page

When asked why he did not write a book about losing weight, a triathlete famously replied, "It would be too short. Just one page: burn more [calories] than you consume. Period."

So it would seem that this weight loss chapter could be very light. But there is more to it than meets the athlete's, or Apneac's, eyes. Just as reversing Apnea involves multiple factors, so does weight loss; and weight loss specific to reversing Apnea is as individual as the Apneac and their own specific OSA problem.

## Weight A Predictor

**Excess weight, especially when carried as fat in the neck, is one of the most decisive predictors for Apnea.**
So, here's one blanket rule: in order to heal Apnea, get the weight off. Period. Why? Apneacs are often overweight and the effects of weight loss on OSA are consistently positive.

What about you skinny Apneacs? Focus for these Apneacs will be on other items causing OSA: deviated septum, polyps, oversized nasal turbinate structures, under-toned necks small jaws and tongue muscles. But as you will learn in this chapter, there may also be diet issues related to inflammation and throat muscle dysfunction that applies to all Apneacs, even the slender.

## An Excellent Argument for Weight Loss to Reduce OSA

A common finding of Apnea studies is that approximately 60-70% of all Apneacs are overweight or obese. Other studies show a direct correlation between the amount of weight lost and the reduction in the severity of the Apnea. For example, a study of nearly 700 randomly selected employed Wisconsin residents showed a direct relationship between weight gain and worsening Apnea.

Summarizing their findings, relative to the Apneac's stable weight, a 10% weight gain predicts an approximate 32% increase in the AHI. This means that just **a 10% increase in weight predicts a 6-fold increase in the odds of developing moderate-to-severe Apnea.** Conversely, just a 10% weight loss predicted a 26% decrease in the AHI: very encouraging.

### *Swedes Cut Down*

For Apneacs in a Swedish study, after one year on a calorie restriction diet, CPAP was no longer (according to their metric of an AHI of 10 or less) needed in 30 of 63 patients (47%), while 6 patients (10%) had total remission of Obstructive Sleep Apnea (AHI of less than 5 events/hour.) This shows that when Apneacs get to their ideal weight, their Apnea improves substantially. Patients who benefited most were those with severe Obstructive Sleep Apnea.

Depending on severity of the Apnea, diet may not eliminate the need for CPAP, but weight loss usually improves the Apneac's experience of even CPAP because the machine can be operated at lower pressures, making it more natural, comfortable, and making sleep easier and more restful.

## Weight Loss Works for OSA

Literally the bottom line, weight loss is especially effective for entry-level OSA sufferers. Those sufferers are often not quite ready for CPAP. Plus, it's not as effective with the more advanced form of OSA, Mixed Apnea, since the Central Sleep Apnea component of the disease is a result of brain irregularities in addition to breathing obstruction. However, the brain and respiratory signals may still benefit from a better diet. So it's tempting to ask, why doesn't every Apneac just lose weight?

# Keys to Apneac Weight Loss

✓ Do it.

✓ Do it healthily.

Although weight loss is nearly as simple as modifying one's diet, **with over 60,000 diet books on Amazon, contradictions abound**; it can be both difficult and confusing to decide on a diet, especially when health is at stake. To make matters worse, we are living in a period where macro trends of the fast food industry, and food choices driven by engineered-to-be-tasty refined food **have led to "the blubberfication of America" – a lifestyle of refined carbohydrates, cable TV and cars**. But for most Apneacs, the math is just dead simple:

*(Lose the Blubber) + (Lower general/specific body inflammation) = Lower the AHI score*

## Don't Wait to Lose Weight

The bottom line is getting the weight off. NOW. **Get to your ideal weight, your fighting weight. How much to lose?**

139

**Think back to your teen years**. Perhaps that is a good target. How to get the weight off? More than any other TOOL, excluding perhaps exercise, weight loss is an individual endeavor requiring persistence. Generally, diets change the mix of calories and percentages of the food groups: carbohydrates, proteins and fats, and aim to improve healthy nutrition.

Of course the healthiest weight loss practices are best, but a morbidly obese Apneac may be smart to consider long-term health a luxury: that fat has to come off now. The issue here is to shed those life-threatening pounds, which are known to exacerbate Apnea, before more damage is done and thereby stop accelerating their health's demise.

So more drastic measures may need to be considered. Studies show AHI scores plummeted when the significant weight loss resulted from lap band surgery, because this procedure limits the calories available to the body and results in large weight loss. The critical point here is that lap band surgery delivers, because weight loss delivers.

## Strangled by Fructose

Nearly all experts agree that we should cut down consumption of refined carbohydrates like white flour used in pizzas or many other popular bread products, and high-fructose corn syrup (HFCS) used (instead of sugar) in manufactured foods like cereals, cookies, sodas, soups, ketchup and other sauces. Refined carbohydrates like flour have 14 calories of sugar (glucose) per tablespoon, which quickly enters the bloodstream, but at least all our cells can – slowly – process glucose. Fructose is different. Fructose can only be processed by the liver, yet "food" manufacturers use 10,000% more HFCS than in 1970, mostly in sodas. Snuck into every corner of the American diet, refined carbohydrates and HFCS have, literally, a stranglehold on every Apneac's throat and cardiovascular health.

# What's a Body to Do? (With Sugars)

The liver tries to mop up excess blood sugar by converting glucose to a form of sugar (glycogen) that can be stored in fat cells. The pancreas releases insulin to try to open fat cells to store glycogen, but most are full and resistant to insulin (a condition defining diabetes). Muscle cells can store 2,000 calories of blood sugars and have to do so when we eat foods high in refined carbohydrates.

## We Ate Our Way Into The Problem; We Can Eat Our Way Out

Human nutrition is also subject to individual genetic makeup, current health, and environment. So, depending on who you are and where you live, your healthy diet may be different than someone else's. Understanding you own body and the stresses you experience will help you to create a diet of foods right for you: and you can cut down on products made with refined flours.

## You Are Full of It: Water!

You can also drink your way out of your overweight problem – with water. Thirst and hunger use the same hormonal alert system in the body, so if you feel hungry after meals, it is likely that your liver is running out of water. By drinking sufficient water, a body that so often felt so hungry, can begin to feel full and regain the ability to absorb nutrients. Then the brain starts getting the "I am full" message.

## All Calories Don't Count The Same

Simply counting calories to lose weight sounds logical. Eat less than you burn. Calories matter. Yet our bodies do not treat all calories in the same way.

Dark chocolate, for instance, contains sugar and fat, but also helps us stay lean because it contains antioxidants (polyphenols) that slow sugar absorption and fat oxidization. (Just don't take this as an excuse to gorge on chocolate.)

Many dark/colored foods like berries (black, blue, purple, red, yellow-orange) are rich in polyphenols that speed weight loss.

# Nice Mangos!

Every day, scientists find new anti-oxidant compounds in fruits, veggies, seeds and herbs that help to lower blood sugar and increase weight loss. A recent discovery touted by Dr. Oz. is an African mango. Sales are soaring!

## Diet of Early Man

All plant and animal foods have "goodies" in them; defense chemicals that inhibit cell breakdown, and also – in raw foods – enzymes that streamline cell turnover. When we digest these plants and animals, we get the benefits of those "goodies." The beneficial "goodies" vary from food to food, and the ability to utilize each "goodie" is an acquired, evolutionary process. Early humans evolved over eons to eat raw enzyme-rich meats, eggs, nuts, seeds, fruit and vegetables: a balanced natural diet. Aside from early humans' short life span due to spear wars with the low-rent Cro-Magnons, and the occasional inconvenience of a mastodon herd stampeding through the extended family Yurt, interrupting Tarzan re-runs, life was good. There were no taxes and no root canals.

Food didn't change until about 10,000 years ago when agriculture began. That made grains, also known as carbohydrates, the staple of our diet. The next dietary change came as we began keeping cattle and eating dairy products about 8,000 years ago. But our genes still haven't caught up with those ancient changes: **30% of us lack effective digestive enzymes to metabolize the wheat and dairy that constitutes the bulk of our modern diets**. Unlike our computers, we cannot simply download a new system patch and process the new diet data. Consequently, our immune systems still react to these "new" proteins as if they were invading bacteria. Then in the last 50 years, things got even worse. The advent of "modern" processed foods threw a batch of monkey wrenches into our metabolic and immune systems.

## Avoidance Eating

Armed with the most basic understanding of our digestive inheritance, there are a few simple concepts that can simplify dieting. There are at least a few foods that we should simply avoiding eating.

### Sneaky High-Sugar Foods

Sneaky high-sugar foods include those you think are healthier than regular food or drink: salad dressings and energy bars, bottled energy drinks, teas and diet sodas, as well as fat-free frozen desserts! Whether "fat-free" or not, ice cream isn't a diet food. Sherbet, too, is not a diet food. Sorry. Manufacturers add

143

sugar to low-fat foods like yogurt and milk, and this increases weight gain, whether the sugars are natural or altered (high-fructose corn syrup) or even supposedly zero-calorie, "non-nutritive" artificial sugar substitutes.

### High-Carbohydrate Low-Fiber Foods

High-carbohydrate low-fiber foods like white potatoes, white rice and white bread fatten you almost as fast as they turn into sugars.

# Sugar Depresses Your Immune System!

Your body's immune system uses white blood cells to destroy viruses and bacteria. In the 1970's, researchers discovered that a lot of Vitamin C was needed by white blood cells to do this. Sugar's chemical structure is similar to vitamin C. As your blood glucose levels increase, glucose competes with vitamin C to enter white blood cells. If there is more glucose present, less vitamin C will enter the cell. Unfortunately, it doesn't take much glucose for this disruption to occur. Normal blood glucose levels after a breakfast of toast with jam, or a sandwich, range from 135-140 milligrams per deciliter, but a blood glucose level of 120 can reduce immune system functioning by 75%. Believe it! When you eat sugar, you depress your immune system!

### Refined Concentrated Proteins

Refined concentrated proteins are another class of foods that an Apneac ought to investigate and probably avoid. Refined concentrated proteins can confuse and stimulate the immune system. Here's why: certain proteins (like gluten in bread, elements of peanuts, or soy protein isolates) can cause food allergies. Allergies are the interaction of immune cells with proteins that they can't identify. Immune cells are intolerant of foreign proteins because they identify them as foreign life, a possible threat.

For example, gluten, which is found in wheat, rye and barley, contains a unique protein, gliadin, that squeezes between cells in the throat or gut, and enters the blood. Immune cells can react to these gluten particles in the blood whenever you eat a bite of wheat bread and this can lead to chronic inflammation. Allergies can cause swelling of airways and this can worsen Apnea.

## Sleep More

Stress studies show that sleeping less than 6 hours impairs the body's ability to regulate blood sugar, and increases the risk of diabetes. This risk also applies to the Apneac's partner, who may not get enough sleep due to the Apneac's snoring.

Added to less sleep, poor diets and less physical activity, and the weight adds up. Sleep makes a big difference. On the same diet, **dieters who slept 8 hours lost 50% more than those who slept only 5 hours**. In our "modern" fast-paced American society, sleep is sacrificed; compared with 50 years ago, Americans are sleeping 1 to 2 hours less per night, and Apneacs and their partners are among the biggest sleep losers.

## Fats You Don't Need

Inflammation is an Apneac's enemy. This means that there are fats that a body should generally avoid. These are mostly modern creations.

## *Trans Fats*

Trans fats (partially hydrogenated oils and margarines) interfere with the body's synthesis of disease-fighting immune T-cells.

## *Polyunsaturated Fatty Acids*

Polyunsaturated fatty acids (PUFAs); these modern processed oils derived from corn and soybean and other vegetables, (safflower and sunflower) seeds, grains, and legumes are high in inflammatory omega-6 fatty acids, provoking allergies.

# No Silver Bullet

One over-arching them of this book is that there is no silver bullet for Apnea. This is especially true for diets – and not just diets for Apneac, but diets for all people. Different strokes for different folks. Some do well with a raw food diet, while others may benefit from a low-fat diet, while still others lose weight with new findings that support high-fat diets. As an Apnea Avenger, this is where your own personal program needs to be stepped-up. You need to do the legwork to find out what works for you.

Get the fat off. Weight loss almost always translates to a reduction of NC (neck circumference). So, the message here is twofold. First, **get the fat off the neck**, lose the fat that causes inflammation. And second, **learn which foods drive general inflammation in your body, and then avoid them**. Fat and inflammation. These are your enemies, Apnea Avengers.

Don't wait to lose weight.

# CHAPTER 9:
# Sweat Your Way to Sleep

## *Tethered to The Grid*

*Over the years, I've been able to adventure around the world. On one trip, my wife and I sailed around the Seychelles with several other couples and one single friend. As I flew from San Francisco, to London, and then on the Nairobi, I began to feel a bit panicky about my snoring. Our boat was small and tight. Would they throw me overboard? Smother me in my sleep? Shoot me with the flare gun? Somehow, it worked out and our friends were either gracious, hard of hearing, or had earplugs and we all survived the trip. A few years later, I committed to treating my Apnea with CPAP. No exceptions. Not until something better came around. Then it happened. One of my adventure buddies from that sailing trip asked if I'd like to hike to the base camp of Everest. Always a dream of mine, I seriously considered it. It was with a heavy heart that I declined. No electricity. No CPAP. Tethered to the grid. There has to be a better way.*

*~W.E.H.*

# The Second System TOOL

In the previous chapter, which we wanted to call Chapter Ate, we went deep into the first TOOL in the System TOOLs drawer: Weight Loss through Diet. In this chapter, we'll develop the other TOOL in the System TOOLs drawer: Weight Loss through Exercise.

# WEIGHT LOSS TOOL: Exercise

## Avoid Sitting to Death

If humanity makes it through global climate change, future historians may be tempted to title this age the "Tsunami of Blubber." Our modern sedentary lifestyle and nonstop spectator entertainments such as sports, TV and video games increasingly remove the population from endeavors that are self-exercise oriented. Even our work is mostly sedentary, and for many, work also involves a computer. **As both individuals and as a nation, we must avoid sitting to death.**

According to an article in the June 2011 issue of the Journal of the American Medical Association, measuring the risks associated with television watching alone, researchers found a direct link between television watching and diabetes, cardiovascular disease, and death. This is not a slight statistical risk, no: for every 100,000 people, excessive television time predicts 104 deaths per year.

## Neurons That Fire Together Wire Together

Far from being hardwired, as scientists once envisioned, the brain is constantly being rewired. The ability of the brain and nervous system to change both structurally and functionally in response to input from one's surroundings is called neuroplasticity. That means the brain is more like clay, more changeable and certainly not mere static thinking matter. Much like a muscle, the brain can be exercised through use, as in learning or thinking. Simply exercising the body can also enhance the brain. **Exercise spawns neurons and the stimulation of environmental enrichment helps those cells survive, but learning combined with exercise creates much bushier, healthier, better-connected neurons**. Neuroplasticity is involved in learning, healing, and with regards to the brain itself, cortical remapping in response to brain injury. Since neuroplasticity is known to improve through exercise, it makes sense that the brain damage that has accrued from acute Apnea may be reversed by a program that utilizes exercise as a control for Apnea.

## Exercise Easy

Start easy. Avoid complications from "overdoing" exercises and developing strained muscles, especially if you have not been following an exercise routine (and this becomes even more important with increasing age). If you are not experienced with exercise, or are "out of shape," or have a medical condition such as Apnea, you would also be wise to seek the guidance of an experienced physical trainer. We also advise you to talk to your doctor(s) before exercising in order to determine which sports or activities best suit your health and physical capabilities.

Exercise speeds the process by which brain cells form connections, causing a "huge increase in the growth factors in the brain," according to Dr. John Ratey, an associate professor of psychiatry at Harvard Medical School, and author of "Spark: The Revolutionary Science of Exercise and the Brain." Dr. Ratey, who has been researching the effectiveness of exercise in treating depression, states unequivocally, "We are talking about seriously ill people here – the clinically depressed. They are responding to exercise." We all know that just one night of sleeping badly is depressing in itself. Research has shown conclusively that long-term untreated Apnea involves brain damage. We also know that when a person decides to employ exercise to reverse brain damage, the performance of more complex exercise tasks leads to much better results.

# Burn More Calories

As was discussed in the previous chapter, there are some exciting developments in our understanding of diet, calories, metabolism, and weight loss. We also talked about Superfoods. Here in the context of exercise, we're going to simplify. Everyday, a certain number of calories get burned, maintaining your base life-sustaining level. This is called the metabolic rate. It's the equivalent to just keeping the lights on. Minimal calories required to digest, to breathe, and to run your heart and power normal daily functions make up this number. Added to that base level are calories to provide energy for exercise, like walking to work. These two components make up the daily energy needs for the day.

Each day, there are calories eaten as a matter of normal life. These vary with most people. When the calories needed and the calories burned are the same, weight is maintained. However, when you eat more calories than you burn in a day, they get stored very easily. When you eat fewer calories than you burn, the body supplements the energy needed to at least meet the base metabolic rate with energy from the body, either by burning fat calories or burning energy stored in the muscles. **Getting the calories burned to come from fat is harder than it is to store fat**. Over time, a regime of eating fewer calories than the body requires can lead to fat loss. Much of it depends on what you eat and how you exercise. Various scenarios of exercise and eating can determine different outcomes of what gets burned during the day, but to an Apneac carrying excess weight around the neck, fat burning is most important. Therefore, how to engage maximum fat burning with exercise and heart rates is covered later in this chapter. First there are critical key things to know when it comes to intensity.

## Workout: Fat Meal First, Carbs After

Eat fat rather than carbs before exercising to improve performance as well as endurance. Fat provides twice the energy needed for heavy exercise and triggers less of an insulin response before a workout, so you're better able to sustain the workout. If you eat carbohydrates before exercising, the high blood sugar will force your body to burn your last meal rather than your fat. So you're less likely to lose weight in this scenario. For instance, do not eat a banana on cereal before exercise; your body will burn the sugary meal instead of fat. Instead, eat an avocado, or a slice of cheese, or a whole milk full-fat yogurt before the workout. Eat a meal with slowly digesting carbs after a workout (not fast sugars like fruit juice), to replenish depleted glycogen stores in your muscles and liver.

After workouts, also eat some protein to help produce the human growth hormone that will keep you lean.

Choose any sport. **Exertion at a moderate-to-high intensity is required to burn the maximum number of calories**. What does that mean," moderate-to-high intensity exertion?" Moderately intensive exercise means that you can talk while playing a sport. Vigorous exercise means you can hardly say more than a few words between breaths. Each minute of vigorous activity or sport is the same as two minutes at a more moderate pace. Yet you can exercise longer at a moderate pace.

So, on the other leg, a much longer, meditative walk would be less impactful while healing on more levels, and would end up burning more calories from fat stores than a more stressful, shorter duration exertion, such as running.

## Systemic Exercise

General whole-body exercise is directly related to the overall reduction of fat tissues in the body. For Apneacs, this often includes a slimming of the neck. This is beneficial to the goal of easing or reducing Apnea. It's a big piece of the larger puzzle.Diet and exercise and fitness books must be among the most popular self-help reference topics, second only to the relationship section where books can be found to help one cope with a romantic break-up, or, worse, divorce. How much failed romance might have been avoided with fitness and a lot less snoring?

# Relationship Satisfaction

Participants of a four-year study often voiced concern that if snoring continued, divorce or separation would result. Sure enough, further research to investigate the impact of snoring on relationship satisfaction confirmed, "Snoring places huge strains on interpersonal relationships." Perhaps most disheartening was to document that 85 percent of snorers typically sleep in other beds in other rooms, alone and apart from their partner.

With our focus on Apnea, we'll discuss exercise in terms of overall health and activity. **Overall health and activity are so closely related that we want you to connect the dots: any improvement of health through exercise will directly correlate to a reduction of NC, a reduction of BMI, and a significant improvement in Apnea scores.**

If the improvement is considerable, Apneacs may find that, for as long as the exercise regimen is continued, there may be a long-term reduction or even elimination of the need for CPAP. But before pitching your CPAP in the closet, confer with your doctor!

### *Movement Tones*

In all forms of exercise, movement is good. Tone comes with movement. So general exercise and fitness toning through yoga, Pilates, walking, jogging, swimming, paddling, weights, dancing, jumping, bouncing and just about all organized sports have to be considered beneficial for the treatment of Apnea. Overall tone and fitness contributes to the tone and fitness of the neck, mouth and tongue muscles, and neck structure – all of which are directly involved in the underlying cause of Apnea.

While exercise, in general, is a beneficial TOOL for the treatment of Apnea, we should first consider how to optimize exercise for maximum benefit. The answer, of course, is at the heart. The key question is: "When exercising, what heart rate is the best to burn fat?"

## Anaerobic Threshold: Maximize Blubber Burning

If you hit the gym, likely you have heard of Anaerobic Threshold (AT), or AT levels. "Dude," they'll say, "Stay below your AT level to get those abs to show." Awareness of **Anaerobic Threshold is THE key to burning fat quickly and first**, which means that this is a key concept for anyone serious about easing his or her Apnea. Apnea Avengers stay on the low side of Anaerobic Threshold.

### Anaerobic Threshold

Anaerobic Threshold (AT) is the maximum heart rate at which the body can operate while continuing to utilize body fat for fuel. It's most easily measured by heart rate. **At higher heart rates, the body switches to more readily available energy, which is sourced from the glycogen, which are sugars stored in the muscles themselves**. Since there is a limited amount of glycogen stored in the muscles, this heart rate cannot be continued for as long.

Even athletes cannot exceed their AT for very long before running out of energy. So just how is AT relevant to non-athletes, to mere mortals? One big step towards healing Apnea is to realize that we are ALL athletes. Apneacs, too, have an AT, and Apneacs, too, can be more or less "out of shape."

**It turns out that you need to be in reasonably good shape just to sleep well**.

So if your goal is to sleep well, then you'll also want to develop an overall healthier and active and productive lifestyle so that you can have a productive life during waking hours.

# Anaerobic Threshold (AT) Simplified

The anaerobic threshold occurs at about 85-90% of maximum heart rate. Your maximum heart rate is easily determined by starting with the number 220 and then subtracting your age. So, for an individual of 30 years age, AT is 85% x (220-30) or 85% of 190, which is 161 beats per minute (bpm). For an individual 55 years old, AT would be 85% x (220-55) or 85% of 165, which is 140bpm. To obtain a more conservative AT and optimize fat loss from exercise, stay below your AT by about 10 to 15 heat beats per minute.

For Apneacs, getting in shape involves the effort to exercise and lower NC (Neck Circumference). This can be more effectively accomplished if we understand the two fundamentals of AT.

- ✓ The first is that **AT changes with age**. That's because, the older a person gets, the lower the heart rate at which the body switches to the anaerobic zone, meaning that weight loss will only occur at lower and lower heart rates.

- ✓ The second is that **we cannot effectively or efficiently reduce fat if we exceed our anaerobic threshold** while exercising.

That's all there is to using AT to your advantage: know the AT for your age, and don't exceed it, unless for short bursts, as in sprinting. And stay 10 to 15 beats below the threshold. The closer you get to AT, the less fat gets burned as the body prepares to switch over to the new fuel.

## Tour de Fats

Let's take a look at Tour de France riders. How can these guys go for almost 30 days all day long and at speeds that mere mortals cannot maintain for even an hour? The answer is FAT. They have trained their bodies to burn fat at a high level of effort. Tour riders know not to exceed Anaerobic Threshold (AT) for long unless they want their physiology to crash. Since most of us are not tour riders, we need to stay away from the AT edge. That's because we have not trained our bodies to burn fat as efficiently at or near the edge of AT – we do better staying well below our AT. For as we approach AT, our percentage of fat burned is less and less until it goes to 0 at AT, and that's when the body begins to burn our muscles' glycogen. Think of it as a hybrid electric car: most hybrids run off electric battery until they're going about 25 MPH, and then the hybrid switches over to gasoline power. It's much the same with the body, which will first run on fat for a long steady slow burn, but with higher demand the body turns to burning the glycogen sugars that are stored in the muscles.

What about mere mortals who don't ride in the Tour de France. How do we exercise in order to work below AT and thereby reduce my BMI, AHI, and NC? And which exercises are best? There are too many considerations to enumerate them in all one book, much less in a chapter section. But there are innumerable comparisons available. For example, as shown in the two tables on the following page, we found research at LiveStrong.com that compares two different exercises, walking and cycling.

| How to compare two exercises for optimal results, adapted for treating Apnea. | | |
|---|---|---|
| | **Walking** | **Biking** |
| Calories? | Burns less calories | Burns more calories as glycogen, not fat |
| Targets obesity & correlated issues? | More efficient at reducing fat, NC, & BMI: more ideal for Apneacs. | Less efficient at reducing fat, NC, & BMI; less ideal for Apneacs. |
| Relieves stress? | Yes | Yes |
| Exercises metabolism & maintains resting heart rate? | Yes | Yes |

| Typical one hour routines compared according to weight | | |
|---|---|---|
| Weight | Walk 3.5 mph burns | Cycle12-13 mph burns |
| 120 lbs | Approx. 207 cal. | Approx. 435 cal. |
| 150 lbs | Approx. 259 cal. | Approx. 544 cal. |
| 180 lbs | Approx. 310 cal. | Approx. 653 cal. |
| 200 lbs | Approx. 345 cal. | Approx. 726 cal. |
| Walk 3-5 days per week, drop 1/3 of a pound. Lost weight is fat? Yes. | | Bike 3-5 days per week, drop 1/2 to one full pound. Lost weight is fat? Not necessarily. |

# Double Loser – Diet & Exercise

High intensity exercise, such as biking, burns a lot more calories than walking, but relies more on energy stored in muscles in the form of glycogen sugar, whereas walking briskly works off of fat stores. Also, high intensity exercise at or above AT forces the body to access the most readily available energy first, usually the most recent carbohydrates eaten, followed second by fat stores. Understanding this is crucial to successfully combining diet with exercise to burn calories in an effective, healthy way. That's because it is necessary to eat properly to support an exercise program, which includes periods of high intensity exercise. Otherwise, a misguided exercise and diet program may lead to the depletion of muscle mass, or even exhaustion and injury. So when the main goal of an exercise routine is to burn fat, you will want to consider how to exercise below the Anaerobic Threshold (AT).

## Track Calories

Use a site like LiveStrong.com or loseit.com to keep track of how you are eating, what you are eating and what combination of fat, protein, and carbohydrates you are consuming. Both are available on mobile smartphones as well. Why have a Starbucks Maple Oat Nut Scone with over 500 calories when you can have their whole milk yogurt with 140 calories? The more you know, the more you track, the lighter you get.

Yes it is true, you lose weight by burning calories, no matter what. Yet **what's even more important than calories is the balance between high-intensity and low-intensity exercise. That's because fat stores, not muscle mass or**

**stored sugars, must be burned in order to lose fat; and low intensity exercise - extended exercise which is below the AT - burns fat stores most efficiently**.

# Use Brown Fat to Burn Calories

Brown fat keeps you warm by burning about 80 calories an hour – 80% more than white fat cells, because brown fat cells have multiple vacuoles filled with fat, while white fat cells have only one vacuole. Until recently, adults were not thought to have much brown fat, just a few ounces in the upper back, on the sides of the neck, between the collarbone and the shoulder, and along the spine, as well as a little brown fat deep in the body around the kidneys. But according to Dr. Kahn, chief academic officer at the Joslin Diabetes Center in Boston, scans of chilled men exposed deposits of brown fat *in their muscles*. And exercise has been shown to increase the brown fat that helps to keep you warm! When you exercise, your muscle cells release a newly discovered hormone, *Irisin*, which may mediate the iron that makes this fat "brown." Irisin can convert white fat cells into brown ones, which in turn burn extra calories when you are cool. Do you want to sleep with the sheets off? Do you want to sleep with the CPAP off? Then exercise. Pick one and do it. That's what Apnea Avengers do. Apnea Avengers exercise regularly at optimum AT to stay warm and sleep cool, and you can too.

## Activities & Sports for Apneacs

The best exercises for Apneacs are ones that:

- ✓ Offer sustained moderate intensity activity below the optimal AT (85%).
- ✓ Best suit the overall goals of reduced NC and BMI.

✓ Best suit the individual's general health.

✓ Offer the least impediments for each individual. (For example, a swimmer without pool should consider walking or biking rather than delaying for that mythical, "someday when I have access to a pool.")

## What Sports Burn?

In order to lose fat and stay in shape, the body must burn more calories than it consumes. Exercise and sports can burn significant calories. **The number of calories you burn depends as much on the intensity level of the sport or activity as it does on your weight and physical capabilities**.

**For optimal health benefits, five hours of moderately intense aerobic activity is recommended each week**. There are many sports and activities that can provide the needed aerobic punch. We've complied a short list of a few obvious choices.

Remember, exercise for health is a choice for health. So if you are going to do things to lose weight and improve your general health, make good choices. Avenging Apnea is a long-term, life saving exercise.

✓ Be consistent.

✓ Choose your exercise wisely.

✓ Choose something you'll look forward to.

Or indulge in several exercises and change your routine through the week: swim three days and walk two. However you choose to exercise, remember, consistency counts.

## *Yoga*

The American Council on Exercise reports that a typical 50-minute hatha yoga session burns approximately 144 calories, while 50 minutes of more intense power yoga or ashtanga burns about 237 calories. That translates to 172 calories burned in an hour of less intense hatha and 284 calories burned during an hour of ashtanga.

## *Swimming*

Swimming is a sport that burns considerable calories. Depending on your weight and physical capabilities, lap swimming can burn between 511 and 763 calories per hour. Different strokes work various muscle groups and, due to the varied intensity of the strokes themselves, burn different amounts of calories. For example, the butterfly stroke may burn up to 900 calories an hour – if one were capable of swimming butterfly, much less that long! But due to its intensity, it may not burn fat, just glycogen.

# Beginning Swimmers

Beginning swimmers find that this low impact sport is really intense, burning 500 calories per hour merely doing the dog paddle or even ... while "just" treading water.

## *Team Sports*

Depending on your weight, physical capabilities and intensity of play, an hour of basketball burns about 847calories, while touch football burns up to 872. Other team and individual sports that consume 500 or more calories in an hour include softball or baseball, squash, rowing and tennis.

## *Winter Sports*

Popular winter sports and activities that burn a high number of calories include skiing, snowboarding and sledding. Cross-country skiing or ice-skating can burn 436 to 544 calories per hour. Other calorie-burning winter sports include downhill skiing, ice hockey, snowshoeing and sledding.

# Work it Off

Get the fat off. Your AHI will go down. A little weight loss has a big impact in reducing the severity of the Apnea, while significant fat loss can reverse or even eliminate Apnea. Work to get to "your fighting weight!" Swedish studies have shown that this can eliminate the need to CPAP for almost 50% of the Apneacs.

Remember to measure your progress. **Measurement over time works**. It's encouraging to see how much you progress. But, there's just one little detail: you have to actually do it.

So exercise your options: lose weight, sleep better, become awesome and buff.

Be an Apnea Avenger.

# CHAPTER 10:
# Specialty Exercises

## *Surgery or Space Mask?*

*At this point in the progression of my affliction, I knew I needed to step up to a new level. I was tired. My dental appliance was not working well. I had two young kids; a demanding dotcom startup, and my exercise program was spotty. Then, I read about a new way to "fix" Apnea by moving the tongue forward. After consulting with doctors and friends, I decided that, rather than feel decidedly "uncool" and "look sick" by sleeping with a mask and tubes, I would go for the surgery. When I look back now I realize how much of it was vanity. I was thinking just bite the bullet and get the "big ass" surgery done. Yes, I was advised that this surgical approach had a seventy percent "cure rate." I erroneously figured I would certainly be on the lucky side and they probably were citing an unoptimistic number to cover their liability. Ironically, the surgery did not work, and I ultimately had to, and still do, wear a mask with tubes to protect myself from all the chronic conditions spawned by untreated Apnea.*

*~W.E.H.*

# Targeted TOOLs

In the previous chapters we've shown that the Apnea Avenger's TOOLbox contains three big drawers with External TOOLs, System TOOLs and Targeted TOOLs. Here, we will talk in depth about the TOOLs in the Targeted TOOLs drawer, which are Exercise TOOLs.

These exercises, are Circular Breathing, Gum-Control, and Yoga. To review, the term "targeted" indicates that these TOOLs are practices for obtaining specific results in specific areas of the body closely associated with Apnea. These Targeted Exercise TOOLs are where Apnea Avengers shine!

## Three Targeted TOOLs

- ✓ Circular Breathing .

- ✓ Playing a musical wind instrument such as the Didgeridoo.

- ✓ Oropharyngeal Exercise.

- ✓ Isometric Gum-chewing (aka Gum Control).

- ✓ Targeted Yoga.

# Circular Breathing

## *Resistance is Not Futile*

Researchers have found significant improvement in AHI scores as well as reduction in Neck Circumference (NC) when Apneacs practiced circular breathing.

## What is Circular Breathing?

Circular Breathing (CB) is a specialized way of breathing used by musicians while playing musical wind instruments. One such instrument is the Saxophone. The specialized breathing technique used while playing the Sax is called Circular Breathing because it enables the breather to create a constant flow of air out through the lips, uninterrupted, sometimes for as long as an hour.

Proficiency in **this technique involves demanding exercise of the tongue, upper and lower neck, and the nose**. Over 30 musical instruments utilize circular breathing as part of the playing technique. Bet you didn't know that Apnea Avengers are musical!

### *From Nose to Lungs*

Throughout this book we've presented an array of puzzle pieces. Taken together, all these pieces reveal a basic theme: **OSA is an airway problem from the nose to the lungs. Simple mechanics and physics are at work. Pinch points can be found anywhere along the airway**.

A narrow air passage through a neck that is out of tone with weak muscles and blanketed with extra tissue can lay down the OSA gauntlet. For too many this unmitigated bummer comes quite early in life.

The addition of a tongue that's disproportionately large for the airway worsens things. And since we sleep horizontally, gravity is added to the mix, pulling on soft flabby tissue to further obstruct a compromised airway. (This explains why some Apneacs, usually the younger ones, can sleep just fine on the side, yet fall into OSA whenever they attempt to sleep on their back.)

## *Gravity is Inescapable*

Gravity is inescapable. Now imagine that you have both a small air passage and a large tongue. Toss in a deviated septum and you might be fit and at your "fighting weight" but still have little room to breathe.

And that's just one or two variations. Infinite scenarios can find their way into your life through the six potential obstruction points that extend from the tip of the nose to the lungs. As noted previously, these are:

✓ Deviated or blocked nasal septum.

✓ Large or inflamed turbinates.

✓ Uvula tissue.

✓ Tongue size too big for cranial structure or mouth box.

✓ Weak, small or damaged pharyngeal throat muscles.

✓ Enlarged tonsils and adenoids.

Many minds have mulled the problem of OSA. With some success, surgeons apply the knife; device makers make clever devices to move jaws, suck tongues forward, or expand nasal breathing passages.

Implant makers slide stiffeners into weak tissue and electrical stimulating wires into the nerves of the tongue. As discussed in previous chapters, these have a place.

But what about music? Does playing music have a place in the treatment of Apnea? The answer is, "Yes."

## Music Power

At some point, musicians applied their artistic brainpower to an Apneac's dilemma. Perhaps it began like this, "You in the in woodwinds department, you sleeping okay? What? Like little babies? ... Huh?" And so the strings section may have begun to think, "**What do the woodwinds have that we don't?**" A few days later, in another dialog, the woodwinds respond to the strings saying, "Can't talk right now, working like a dog keeping this circular breathing going. My tongue is cramping and my neck is tired." The proverbial light bulb was illuminated. And so we pose the question: Circular breathing. Is it a key? Can such a simple targeted exercise be a TOOL to open the Apneac's airway and even help it to defy gravity?

## An Orchestral Survey

Certain wind instruments require Circular Breathing to deliver a continuous sound. **Great players develop tremendous strength in unusual places, like the throat, neck and tongue**. From an Apneac's point of view these are the most desirable locations for specific targeted exercise. How lucky is this? Very fortunate indeed! Among wind players, the very same musculature implicated in OSA gets an Olympic workout. It all sounds promising, and it is.

A study was conducted to survey over 800 musicians, including conductors, all stripes of instrumentalists, even vocalists. The average age of all participants in the study was 42.5. This is interesting because Apnea is known to worsen with age, which meant the study participants were at their moment of greatest exposure to the disease. Analyzing all of the data, the researchers concluded that, **"naturalistic respiratory muscle training with high resistance wind instruments may reduce risk for OSA in at-risk populations."** Furthermore, they found that risk for OSA was the lowest among the double reed players. The double reed players work their breath long and hard. The researchers also observed that, among these players, the number of hours practiced per week was the most important variable in lowering risk for OSA. Here's the bottom line: duration of play, combined with a high resistance instrument and using Circular Breathing (CB), can lower OSA scores. Lower OSA scores indicate an abatement or reversal of Apnea. A Swiss medical study confirmed the findings of the woodwind survey. Their study focused on the use of CB with a unique high-resistance instrument, the didgeridoo. Playing this eclectic instrument was shown to "significantly" lower the participants' AHI index. Apnea Avengers should do didgeridoo!

### Ok, What's Significant?

Playing for less than 30 minutes a day over a three-month period, the AHI of the didgeridoo players was improved by nearly 40%. As you might expect, the Swiss were thorough. Armed with their army knives, they factored for weight loss, and compared the didgeridoo players to a control group of OSA sufferers.

### Targeted Exercise Delivers Significant Results

Targeted exercise is a TOOL that delivers significant results. **When you can't breathe, an improvement of nearly 40% is important**: especially when that improvement comes from a practice that is as simple (and potentially enjoyable) as playing music on a wind instrument a mere 30 minutes a day.

# Every Healing is Unique

Depending on oral-cranial makeup, not every one will benefit the same. This applies to the didgeridoo as much as to CPAP or any other TOOL that we might try for the treatment and possible reversal of Apnea. Individual differences in physiology as well as lifestyle choices, point to the absolute need for the Apneac to assess all of the pieces of the puzzle, to leave no option unexplored.

Practicing CB is not an invasive, risky, permanent surgery. It's not like training for a marathon. It's just a brief daily interlude for practice. But a word of caution: continue maintenance treatment with CPAP until you can confirm, 100%, that your Apnea has been resolved. You may find that CPAP may still be necessary, but can be adjusted to reflect partial healing. **Remember, healing is a process**. Work at it, but give it time and don't give up trying. Victims give up. Apnea Avengers are relentless in their drive to learn, heal, adjust; they continue learning and adjusting and healing evermore.

## What Circular Breathing Looks Like

Just what does Circular Breathing look or feel like? We found this description from a musician, explaining how he teaches CB: "By blowing bubbles in a beverage with a straw, you can sit around and practice circular breathing for hours while you read or watch TV. But as an oboist, I recommend that you pinch the straw with the fingers so that the opening is more like an oboe reed. Work at it.

Gradually you will find that you can keep the bubbles going through an entire episode of your favorite TV show. When you can go for an hour without a conventional breath, you're more than ready to try it out on the oboe." This bubble method provides great feedback to the breather: when you do Circular Breathing (CB) correctly, the stream of bubbles is continuous. If you miss a breath, the bubbles stop. It's that simple.

## How is CB Physically Accomplished?

The goal of Circular Breathing (CB) is to sustain a constant stream of air traveling out past your lips (or through a straw, or reed, or orifice of a musical instrument) for a long period of time, yet while breathing in and while breathing out. This breathing in and out is accomplished by opening and closing the throat while pushing air out continuously with a bellows action of the cheeks and the tongue.

The technique requires some resistance, thus the straw or pursed lips. When playing woodwind instruments, the resistance is provided by a special mouthpiece called a reed; when playing the didgeridoo, resistance is provided by your vibrating lips.

Imagine using your body like a compressor (which is just an air pump) with two tanks of unequal sizes. The big tank is connected to a second much smaller tank. In your body, the lungs are the big tank, while the bellows action of the mouth, tongue and inflated cheeks form the small tank. Got the picture?

Ok, here's how it works: the small tank, your mouth, tongue and cheeks, has a hose or a small opening where the air is pushed out at a constant flow. That's where the lips meet the musical instrument or the straw.

When the smaller tank starts to lose pressure the bigger tank fills it up again. Since the goal is to have a continuous air flow exiting the hose, or lips, the lungs need to refill the smaller reservoir to keep the flow going.

Of course, there is the catch. Your body has only one air passage! Unlike an air compressor that sucks air in one end and pushes it out the other, when the human body performs Circular Breathing, both the in-flow and out-flow share one air passage. No problem, people are smart, and we have neck muscles and cheeks and we are able to learn coordinated activities. This is how CB is coordinated: when the lungs need more air, we use the muscles in the neck and throat to close off the back of the throat, letting air come down from the nostrils to fill the large tank, your lungs.

While that is happening, we allow the elastic nature of our cheeks to transition from being puffed up and filled with air to now slowly squeezing that air out through the lips at a constant rate. We coordinate this so that the cheeks (small tank) become depleted of air just as the lungs (large tank) are completely refilled with air from the in-breath.

At this point, we relax the back of the throat and allow air to flow back into the mouth, then the cheeks are puffed back up, and a continuous stream of air flows out through the mouth and lips, until the cycle is repeated. This Circular Breathing technique enables the performer to maintain a consistent stream of air, without varying the amount or pressure, flowing endlessly across the lips. Some report that they can do this for hours at a time. CB delivers a constant tone in the instrument and world-class neck muscles.

So how and what does this do for Apnea? **The key factors are the Circular Breathing itself and the amount of resistance while blowing. Combined, those two variables make can render a successful reduction of Neck Circumference.** The longer it's done the more it works. More resistance means more toning of the neck and throat.

Like Gold's Gym 101, when you get a good work out you see results. Do a consistent workout and you stay in shape. It's the same for your neck and tongue. While a six-pack of great abs might seem more impressive, for someone who is determined to become an Apnea Avenger, world-class neck muscles will get you there.

171

# Three-Way Crossing: NC, Tone, and Neural Connection

If Apnea could be depicted with a road map, we'd draw a big red circle around the intersection of Neck Circumference, Neck Tone (or rigidity), and Neural Connections. And we'd send our squad cars there to apprehend the killers who lurk there, OSA and snoring. As was discussed in earlier chapters, **long-term oxygen starvation from Hypopnea and Apnea is thought to be implicated in damaging specific connections to the brain that are responsible for proper muscle tone in the airway**. Research has found that a simple throat virus can damage the nerves in the same region of the airway, leading to numbness and damaged connections.

Harmonizing those two observations, it appears that either one, or even both problems together, result in under-toned muscles that can lead to a narrowing or even a complete obstruction of the airway during asleep. And, although there are many factors at play, this evidence has led researchers to understand that strengthening and toning tongue and the neck muscles makes a difference: **strengthen an Apneac's tongue and neck and you will be likely to see an improvement in the severity of their Apnea**. Muscle tone differs from muscle strength principally in that tone is a function of neural connections. Muscles and nerves are said to be plastic, which means that the level of tone and fitness is never "stuck." Muscles and nerves respond to exercise and can be strengthened, improved, and made more elastic and lively. Lucky for us, the human brain has plasticity, too. Research has shown that **we exercise the related areas of the brain when we exercise specific parts of the body**, and that nerves can be restored and new neural connections can be built by exercising areas of the body where a neural deficit has occurred.

Now we are at the intersection that we circled in red! Circular Breathing (CB) appears to accomplish all three at once: it helps to reduce Neck Circumference while also strengthening and toning the muscles of the neck, throat, and tongue, plus it rejuvenates the related neural connections in the brain. Circular Breathing:

- ✓ Helps reduce Neck Circumference.

- ✓ Strengthens and tones the muscles of the neck, throat, and tongue.

- ✓ Rejuvenates related neural connections in the brain.

### Do More

To begin with, Circular Breathing (CB) is somewhat obscure. To those around us, it may even sound like doing nothing, since it sounds like bureaucrats going around in, well, circles – which can be hard for the rest of us to make time for. Who will take you seriously when you have your calendar open and you say, "Hmmm ... Tuesday, Thursday and Sunday late afternoons are out. I've got Circular Breathing." You get the picture.

## Zen Breathing Room

Confronted by his disciples, a Zen monk was taken to task for multi-tasking. He had been seen at a café, eating breakfast while reading the morning paper. "Master," they implored, "You tell us to have a focused mind. You tell us we must do one thing with concentration and do that one thing only. So how is it that you are seen eating and reading the paper?" "Very simple," the master admonished, "When eating breakfast and reading the paper, eat breakfast and read paper only."

In our multitasking world, doing two things is always better than doing just one. In the same way that going for a long run while listening to music helps to make the run pass more smoothly, it's far more preferable to actually play a musical instrument to get your Circular Breathing done. Plus, it saves on drinking straws. In fact, not only is playing music far less boring, for many it's pretty darn interesting. Of course, many people do not describe themselves as musical and even reject the notion that they can learn to play music. They cite the mechanics of making music as being complicated enough. Overwhelming to many. They say the reality of reading music requires a musical education and that's beyond what they are willing to do. Would we rather suffer for years and die early? Not the Apnea Avengers. They know of a better, cooler, more effective way. Fear not! Enter the didgeridoo!

# The World's Coolest, Easiest Musical TOOL

"Whoa," You say, "Isn't that the ethnic sound coming from that long hollow tube?" Yes. That would be the didgeridoo. And that, too, is the good news. This particular instrument, the didgeridoo, is excellent for an Apneac without musical training! Here's the YES list:

✓ It has only one note. Yes, one note. The length the didgeridoo determines what note it emits; the longer the tube, the lower the note. Nothing more to do.

✓ No sheet music is involved. One note, remember? No finger holes, no strings. No keys. Nothing to fret. Yet that one note opens a world of variation and creativity. With little effort, that one note can be bent and manipulated by the lips and tongue. And since the instrument vibrates when played properly, it's played by ear and feeling, often with eyes closed. Remember the 60's?

✓ It's meditative. Start getting that good vibration, and it resonates at the same frequencies that refresh our human brains when relaxed or meditative.

✓ No animals are ever harmed in the making or use of any didgeridoo.

### Buns of Steel for Your Shoulders?

What single activity can deliver a strong, toned neck, and a Neck Circumference that's more alluring to your mate than the proverbial "buns of steel?" That's right, didgeridoo-ing. In fact, the signature "drone" of the didgeridoo requires the movement of a significant volume of air; so playing exercises complex coordinated breathing between the tongue, cheeks, upper airway, throat and lower diaphragm. It's therapeutic for the brain, the muscles, the mood and overall motivation. And it's comforting for your kangaroo, too.

## Didgeridoo-ology

Thought to be the longest undisturbed culture, dating back 40,000 years, the aboriginal tribes in Australia have been using this ancient instrument, the didgeridoo, for at least 2,000 years. It isn't clear just how the goofy name, didgeridoo, came about. You might think it's aboriginal, but it's not. Thought to be derived from an Irish name, the *Didgeridoo* is reported to have been named in the 1920's by Herbert Basedow, an Australian explorer and friend of the aboriginal culture. Depending on the tribe, local aboriginal names are numerous, with an estimated forty-five variants.

Traditional didgeridoos are found, not made. They are found at the intersection of termites, rotten logs and outback wanderings. This makes them quite rare. Traditional players find a branch that has been hollowed out in the center by termites, take it home, clean it up, then cut it to length for the desired note and sound.

Men play the didgeridoo. Traditionally, this is how they make a connection with their spirits and dreamtime. It's the bridge. Women don't play because in more evolved cultures, it's understood that women are already connected. Now the didgeridoo can be a bridge to better health for any Apneac.

Modern didgeridoos are manufactured out of acrylic, plastic, metal, bamboo, agave plants or even glass. For about five dollars, a pleasant sounding didgeridoo can be made from a length of PVC pipe. They can also be had for thousands of dollars made from ceramic glass. Surprisingly, the five-dollar version sounds very close to the concert quality glass.

Playing this instrument is often associated with meditation. Why is the didgeridoo felt to be meditative? The sound of the didgeridoo extends down into the very low frequencies, even below Alpha. Alpha waves with a frequency of 8-12 Hz, which correlate to a mental state of rest and focus, yield increased capabilities for creativity. Going lower to 4-7 Hz for Theta waves and even down to 3-0.5 Hz for Delta waves, is where states of well-being are "realized." These low frequency waves reside in roughly the same range as the rhythmic drumming commonly found in the music of indigenous peoples all over the world. The extremely low frequencies are produced by interference between two close frequencies: one from the harmonics, the other from the vocal cords. Those two combine and create low overtones that many players and listeners find restful. The combination is often described as inducing altered states of mind.

Contemporary, local players report that the rhythmic, low frequency harmonics combined with the breath work of playing both relaxes and helps clear the mind.

Think about the benefits of heavy breathing. Now would also be a good time to think of your mate. We mean the motivation of sleeping with your mate instead of alone and strapped to the air hose of your CPAP. Now think about the benefits of heavy breathing on a body's oxygen saturation. No matter what you are thinking now, one thing is sure about the didgeridoo: it sure can't hurt.

# Effective Bubble Therapy TOOL for Circular Breathing

Earlier in this chapter we described the use of a straw and a glass of water to demonstrate circular breathing. We noted there that this method provides excellent feedback: seeing a constant stream of bubbles coming out of the straw confirms CB is being performed correctly. So here's an effective bubble therapy TOOL for Circular Breathing. Although convenient and small, the straw and glass lack sufficient resistance to provide significant therapy in strengthening the airway and tongue. The simple solution? Supersize.

Supersize the straw by replacing it with a simple four foot long, two inch diameter section of PVC pipe; supersize the water glass by replacing it with a water bucket. Both are available at Home Despot. If you are fortunate enough to have a hot tub or swimming pool, go outside and dip in your didgeridoo. (In addition to your hands, you can use your bare feet to grasp the didgeridoo on either side to prevent it from dropping into the water.)

## *Blowing It*

Now you're ready to work out. The water provides good therapeutic resistance; that steady stream of bubbles assures that you're doing it correctly. Do this twenty-five minutes per day. For more resistance, lower the tube deeper in the water. If you can't be outside by the pool watching the clouds and birds go by, you could relax in front of the TV. Bubbling like this is nearly silent and provides an easy alternative to playing a musical instrument. Just be careful that a family member doesn't kick the bucket.

# Oral Facial Toning Exercise

Intuitively, the idea of a workout for the mouth and tongue make sense, but how?

### Resistance Training for The Airway

Targeted exercise is one of the primary TOOLs to treat and possibly reverse Apnea. Without being too tongue-in-cheek, we'd suggest that the ideal targeted exercise would improve the muscle fitness in the same area where the throat is collapsing. While every Apneac may not dream of being a didgeridoo musician, it still might be good to have a dream. And no one gets to dreamtime without sleep. So with this in mind, what are the alternatives to the didgeridoo? What TOOLs or targeted exercises have been "shown to work in a medical study" for the treatment of Apnea?

### An Argument for Oral-Facial Exercises

Oropharyngeal exercise for pharyngeal fitness: yes, we know, this sounds like a science fiction sub-species. But oropharyngeal refers to the tongue and air passage, or throat. Saying the word is an exercise in itself, for it seems to be more easily stuck in the mouth than uttered. Perhaps that's good, because oropharyngeal exercise is just medical-speak for exercising the tongue and throat.

## Speaking of Tongues

Human tongues are much bigger than what we see. The tongue is like the tip of the iceberg. In fact, the whole tongue is about the size of both fists pushed together. Often referred to as the strongest muscle(s) in

179

the body, the human tongue is made up of eight muscles. Extraordinary strength is attributed to the tongue because words that it forms can sometimes move mountains and pyramids. Yet from an Apneac's perspective, the tongue can be the deadliest muscle. For Apnea is often driven by a weak tongue or one that's too big for it's own good; a flaccid tongue flopped to the back of the throat to obstruct the sleeper's airway, minute-after-minute, hour-after-hour, night-after-night. Such a tongue can kill the biggest and strongest body.

The subjects of medical studies, oropharyngeal isometrics and isotonic exercises have been shown to produce significant lowering of the Apnea-hypopnea Index (AHI). As with all exercise, practice makes perfect. So in this case perfect is, again, getting the equivalent to six-pack abs, but in the tongue's case it's an eight-pack because you have eight big muscles in that deceptively small tongue.

## An Innovative Medical Study in Brazil

A pivotal, innovative medical study measuring the success of a targeted-exercise approach for the treatment of Apnea was conducted in Brazil. The research team was at the Sleep Laboratory, Pulmonary Division, Heart Institute (InCor), at the University of São Paulo Medical School, in São Paulo. In this study, a daily exercise routine was given to thirty-one patients with moderate OSA, for a three-month period. The routine included sixteen exercises aimed at the tongue, soft palate, and lateral pharyngeal wall. Did they get good results? **AHI scores were reduced from 22 to 14 events per hour! Even oxygen saturation improved. Additionally, Neck**

**Circumference (NC) was reduced**. That alone is significant news for Apneacs seeking pieces of the puzzle because it's known from other research that any change in NC results in a likely improvement of Apnea symptoms.

Furthermore, weight change was shown not to factor in the results; there was no significant change in either BMI (body mass index) or abdominal circumference. In their findings, the researchers noted that the participants would need to continue the exercises in order to get the results.

Although the study group is considered statistically small, the results are encouraging for Apnea Avengers, because in targeting the NC – lower the NC and you can lower the AHI – the logic for a pro-active treatment and possible healing of Apnea is advanced.

## Easier Targeted Exercises

The targeted-exercise routine used in the Brazilian study was complex and required the regular engagement of the researchers throughout the three-month period in order to keep the participants on track. It also required a substantial daily time commitment as well as a degree of learning. Our observation? It must have been hard to keep going on that program. (If you are interested, we've included the exercise descriptions, in their entirety, in the Citations Appendix at the end of the book.)

To work **in modern society, the success or failure of an exercise routine may hinge on it being easy enough and convenient enough that the exercise can be integrated into daily life** (especially a routine to exercise the face). To solve this, we were literally inspired by the Brazilian exercises to create a hybrid targeted-exercise TOOL that leads the Apneac through a routine of the sixteen exercises. We call this routine "Gum-Control." And all you need to remember is this mnemonic: "So Breathe"

181

# Practicing Gum-Control

We know human nature. It's easier to take a pill, have a surgery, or even do nothing than to establish a healthy routine for yourself, even if that routine is aimed at tossing OSA on its proverbial butt. But there is no magic bullet to reverse OSA; based on the complexity of the disease, a magic bullet isn't likely, either. Some surgeries work for some. And CPAP doesn't heal or reverse Apnea. Importantly, though, it does stop OSA while you wear it: but only when it's being worn. And certainly not when it is forgotten. For a reversal of OSA, however, what might be easier than chewing gum? Gum is fun to chew and, as shown in the Brazilian study, targeted oropharyngeal exercises work. How about combining the two?

## Isometric Chew

We knew we wanted a purposeful, targeted, isometric and toning gum-chewing regimen. **A mastication plan is an exercise routine, calisthenics for the mouth, that works out targeted areas which, when weak, flabby, or at a loss for tone, are often implicated in Apnea**. We knew that, combined with a mastication plan, chewing is where the action is. Simple as it seems, **purposeful gum chewing can reduce snoring and OSA**. Just don't confuse this with everyday, easygoing gum chewing; this is targeted-exercise. It's "Gum-Control."

## Chew On This

As far as treats go, chewing gum may be older than any other candy. Prehistoric people enjoyed chewing tree resin. Ancient Greeks chewed what they called "mastiche," which consisted of lumps of mastic tree resin. (Texts tell that they enjoyed it and it refreshed their breath as it helped clean their classical smiles.) Native Americans chewed sap from trees, and early American settlers chewed tree sap mixed with beeswax, which made the mixture softer. But it wasn't until 1848 when an entrepreneur introduced gum "for-sale." It was called "State of Maine Spruce Gum." In 1871 another entrepreneur introduced modern gum and patented it. His gum was "Adams New York No. 1." He then followed it with a flavored version, "Black Jack," which can still be found at candy counters. But it wasn't until fifty years later that gum really began to stick; in 1906 Frank Henry Fleer offered the first bubble gum; it had a pretty catchy name, "Blibber-Blubber."

Just so you know, "Gum-Contol" is serious business. You won't take our gum away unless you pry it out of our cold, dead hands. And, as Apnea Avengers, we intend to be kicking and chewing here for a good long while. Purposeful chewing can and should be tiring. We recommend that you use five sticks. Not just one, that's for rank amateurs.

The five-stick regimen is Olympic Chewing. It provides the necessary resistance to give your tongue a perfect eight-pack. It separates the Apneacs from the Apnea Avengers. Add to this, your purpose: healing. Twenty-five minutes of heavy Gum-Control is simple, but it's not easy. Done right, your tongue hits the wall.

Gum-Control can be practiced every day. The average work commute in the USA is twenty-five minutes, which is exactly enough time. Don't want other drivers you don't know (and likely never will) to see you chewing purposefully? Wear shades. Or Practice Gum-Control while plopped in front of the TV. Everyone in modern society multi-tasks, so just learn to chew purposefully along with something else that you do! Just do it daily.

Will Gum-Control address all forms of Apnea? No. But it will address at least one of the six OSA obstruction points in the body, the tongue. It also helps tone the throat. But if you've been told your Apnea is driven by a deviated septum in your nasal passage, gum control won't be effective in reversing that. That said, Gum-Control is a good TOOL and it's easy to use. Just don't use a screwdriver to address a nail.

## What Does Purposeful Mean?

The Gum-Control approach integrates key exercises from the oropharyngeal isometrics and isotonic study conducted in Brazil with a large wad of five-sticks of gum for substantial resistance. Everyday recreational chewing is chewing one stick of gum while moving the tongue around. This can be done all day long – and lots of people do.

Purposeful chewing, or Gum-Control, is chewing with a load of five sticks for resistance because it's associated with a goal. In gym-speak, it's resistance and repetition. The goal is to **exercise your tongue while chewing so that, by the end of your daily practice, the tongue is tired out**. Like after a good long run, it can sometimes be awkward to walk, well, after a good purposeful chew, it could even be difficult to talk. How else are you gonna get a toned eight-pack of tongue muscles?

## The Right Stuff

The right gum makes a big difference. Too soft and it provides too little resistance. Too hard and it's difficult to push around. So,

184

like Goldilocks, you'll want to experiment. (Use sugarless. All moms insist.)

Just as athletes at the gym need to increase their weights, as you get your mouth into better and better shape, you'll add more sticks of gum, or harder gum, so that you'll have something substantial to work with.

But to begin with, three to five sticks are good. Bubble gum has the advantage that you can separate it with your tongue, push it around, and ... blow bubbles.

In order to make Gum-Control easy, we've created a simple two-word phrase, or mantra, to help it the sequence stick in your mind: S-O-B-R-E-A-T-H-E.

# S-O-B-R-E-A-T-H-E GUM CONTROL TOOL

The targeted-exercise Gum-Control TOOL shown in the table on the following 3 pages will lead you through this routine. As with exercises at the gym, there is the exercise itself and there is the number of repetitions. Both are important. The routine is also important: it begins at the top of the mouth and works through all the muscles as it progresses to the bottom of the mouth. So if you are serious about kicking OSA, grab your Juicy Fruit and a towel, slip five sticks of gum in your mouth, turn up your favorite tunes and get your chew on. Apnea Avengers have the taste bud physique of a Greek god. Make the next twenty-five minutes count. End your routine tired. As with all exercise programs or routines, consistency is the key

## S-O-B-R-E-A-T-H-E

### Gum-Control: So Breathe

| | Name | Description | Reps |
|---|---|---|---|
| S | Suck Ups | ✓ Suck tongue up into the roof of the mouth.<br>✓ Hold it there for a count of 20. | |
| O | Over Curls | ✓ Slide tongue up against the roof of the mouth, moving it from behind the front upper teeth to the back of the throat.<br>✓ Keep up the pressure against the upper palate. | 20 |
| | | *By now the tongue should be getting tired.*<br>*The exercise works all eight muscles in the tongue.* | |
| B | Bubble Extensions | ✓ Extend tongue as far out as possible and hold.<br>✓ Hold it there for 10 seconds. | 20 |
| | | *Roof Press is done at 80% resistance, with a good solid hold in each position.* | |
| R | Roof Press | ✓ Push gum to the left side of the jaw and press.<br>✓ Push gum to the right side of the jaw and press. | 20 |
| | | *The Brazilian study included facial exercises. This is the best.* | |

| | | |
|---|---|---|
| E | Eye Raises | ✓ Raise the left cheek up to the eye and hold.<br>✓ Raise the right cheek up to the eye and hold.<br>✓ Hold each side for 10 seconds at 80% effort. | 10 |

*This exercise works the jaw and associated muscles.*
*The concept here is to slide the jaw from side to side.*

| A | Alternate Mastication | ✓ Chew gum on each side of your mouth twenty times.<br>✓ Right side: twenty chews.<br>✓ Left side: twenty chews. | 5 |

*Sports fans know this one. Hit the ball and let out a grunt.*
*It's good for the toning the airway muscles.*

| T | Tennis Grunt | ✓ Imagine that you are dead lifting a heavy weight or smashing a tennis ball.<br>✓ GRUNT. | 20 |

*This exercise will reengage the tongue with a circular rotation.*

| H | Heavy D (BIG rapper who died) | ✓ Press the tongue up against the right side of the upper hard palate.<br>✓ Then press up against the left side of the upper hard palate.<br>✓ Then press down against the right lower teeth and jaw.<br>✓ Then press down against the left lower teeth and jaw.<br>✓ Repeat the circle. | 10 |

*Final exercise: stick your tongue out and move it side to side.*
*Push the gum out like bubble-blowing to increase the resistance.*

| | | 20 |
|---|---|---|
| **E** | Extensions (side slide) | ✓ Take the gum and push through it, extending your tongue out as far as it goes - like blowing a bubble.<br>✓ Swing tongue to the left.<br>✓ Reset.<br>✓ Chew.<br>✓ Take the gum and push through it, extending your tongue out as far as it goes - like blowing a bubble.<br>✓ Swing tongue to the right. |
| | Repeat | *When you finish with "E" pause for a minute or two of random chewing, then repeat the routine. Continue to repeat the entire routine for 25 to 30 minutes.* |

*30 minutes? Ok, you're through. Take a breath to chill that chew.*

## Gums With Benefits

Various gums come with various claims. Green tea gum is said to be good for the body due to its antioxidant content. Hoodia gum, native to the semi-deserts of South Africa, Botswana, Namibia and Angola is hyped as an appetite suppressor, although medical doctors disagree. Cinnamon is known to improve insulin acceptance at the receptor level and lower resistance, so gum infused with cinnamon might be helpful, but may lack adequate dosage to do much. Experiment. Try many kinds and decide what works.

# YOGA

### Yoga Can Provide Targeted Training

We have scant "official" medical research proving that Yoga provides any specific benefit to Apneacs. But the global benefits of Yoga are widely recognized and accepted by many – both in and out of medicine – so **why not a Yoga routine for Apnea Avengers seeking mental fitness, healthy breathing, and muscle tone?**

Here are just a few key points that argue both the global and specific benefits of Yoga to improve the health of Apneacs, while possibly contributing to other therapies that halt or even reverse Apnea.

✓ Mental fitness or well-being comes from being fit. Most yoga practices are balanced on what is referred to as the Mind-Body-Spirit triangle. Yoga may not appeal to every person's taste, but it does have a place for Apnea Avengers. Why? Because **maintaining "a yoga practice" is a workout. Reversing the ravages of untreated OSA is a workout**.

✓ The cornerstone of Yoga is breath. Yet OSA is totally at odds with breath. Yoga celebrates breath, **"You can live for many days without food; you can live for a few days without water; but you cannot live more than a few minutes without breath."** That's how Yoga puts breathing into perspective. It's not just important. It's imperative. So breathing consciously and well through the practice of Yoga is a worthwhile goal.

✓ Breathing and oxygenating the body correlates with and reinforces the goal of halting the advance of Apnea, while possibly helping to reverse it. Why? Because it is the insidious nature of OSA to disrupt the blood-oxygenation, all night long, night after night, week-after-week, year-after-year. This has an incalculable toll on the body. Prior to diagnosis and treatment, the Apneac has suffered constant oxygen deficits bearing damaging insults to the brain and the body. Intuitively, any solid oxygenation – inspiration and expiration – regimen makes sense. Yoga puts this into practice.

✓ Improvement in muscle tone comes from movement and mind-control. As the boys say, "Use it or lose it." Think about it. Yoga is based in movement. Movement enhances muscle tone. Since OSA problems occur mostly in and around the neck, doesn't it make sense that a Yoga regimen could offer poses specifically targeted to exercising the neck? The answer is, "Yes."

Taken together or individually, the following neck-specific yoga poses – named the Camel, Panting Dog or Breath of Fire, Roaring

Lion, Buzzing Bee, and Sun Moon Breathing – comprise another set of Targeted TOOLs for Apnea Avengers to avenge themselves against the killer OSA. It may be a stretch, but Apnea Avengers are down with yoga.

### *Camel*

The Camel pose expands and stretches the chest and abdominal regions. It's excellent for the respiratory and circulatory systems. The pose stretches and strengthens the shoulders and neck, as described below. The Camel pose also activates and balances the Throat Chakra, according to yogic tradition, and works to heal and rejuvenate the thyroid and parathyroid glands in the throat. What are the physical benefits of balancing the Throat Chakra, the fifth of eight Chakras? And what are Chakras?

## Eight Chakras

There are eight chakras in Yoga. These are: the Root Chakra (ovaries or prostate), Sacral Chakra (last [tail] bone in the spinal cord), Solar Plexus Chakra (navel area), the Throat Chakra (neck and throat), Third Eye Chakra (pineal gland), and the Crown Chakra (top of head).

Of the eight chakras, the Throat Chakra is most directly connected with the potential for yogic improvement of OSA. According to yoga teachings, ailments such as a sore throat, mouth ulcers, scoliosis, swollen glands, thyroid dysfunctions, voice problems, gum or tooth problems, and TMJ are connected to the Throat Chakra.

By creating balance at this Throat Chakra, specific areas of the body can also be helped, including the throat, thyroid, trachea, neck vertebrae, mouth, teeth, gums, esophagus, parathyroid glands, and even the hypothalamus (in the brain).

### Do The Camel

Here's how to do the Camel: start by sitting up on your knees with your heels pressed against your buttocks and your shins flat against the floor. Once you're settled, reach back and grab the left ankle with your left hand, then grab your right ankle with your right hand. Breathe in through both nostrils and lift your butt off your legs as you arch your back and push the belly forward, tilting the head as far back as possible. Hold this pose for the duration of one inhaled breath; if you want to hold the Camel pose longer, just breathe gently through the nostrils while holding the posture.

## Panting Dog or Breath of Fire

Breath of Fire is a sophisticated exercise involving breath control. Yogi Bhajan, who was regarded in the west as a mainstream spokesperson for the benefits of yoga, is said to have taught that a person is granted a determinate number of breaths from birth till death. The yogi's logic leads to this: **If you have a predetermined number of breaths in life, make them count.** Use a breath that is good for you, a breath that helps you release tension by moving the diaphragm in and out, that assists in circulation by oxygenation, and also works the breathing muscles. This pose can benefit an Apneac simply by improving OSA symptoms. Like the name indicates, Panting Dog involves, well... panting.

### Panting on Fire

Sit on your shins and lean forward. Now pant through either your nose or mouth. Make sure that the diaphragm is doing the work. Breathe in and out, rapidly. Aim for one to three breaths per second, which is about 120 to 180 times per minute. If you breathe through the mouth, extend your tongue for the best dog-like pant. This targeted-exercise works the diaphragm, which is so critical for healthy breathing.

## Roaring Lion

In everyday life we rarely do such extreme contortions of the exact areas of the body that are both implicated and responsible for OSA. Enter the Roaring Lion. This loud (and under-appreciated-by-the-neighbors) exercise **benefits parts of the body that most other yoga postures do not: the face, jaw, mouth, throat and tongue**. The muscles and tissues of the face are worked out by the alternation of stretching and releasing.

On the 1-to-10 scale, among the Apnea Avenger's weapons to halt or reverse OSA, the Roaring Lion pose rates a solid 10. Did we mention it is loud?

### Just Roar

The Roaring Lion pose is simple. While sitting on your shins, stick your tongue out as far as you can and roar like a lion for a minute. Now repeat that ten times. ROAR.

## Buzzing Bee

The theory for including this targeted exercise with the Apnea Avenger's weapons is that **it strengthens and conditions the pharyngeal wall of the airway**, and may help to protect from OSA collapse. Still, humming like a bee with fingers in your ears? Mmmm. Can it get any weirder? Well, there is a fine line between eccentric and weird. Since you've read this far, our guess is that you're going with eccentric, too.

### We Bee Buzzin"

To do the Buzzing Bee pose, sit on the floor or in a chair, with your legs in front of your body. Take a few breaths in and out.

193

Then, with you lips tightly closed and an index finger in each ear, inhale via the nostrils and then exhale while making the sound of the letter "M." Mmmmmmmmmmmm. Sounds like a buzzing bee. Oh honey, keep making that buzzing noise! Do this for as long as it feels good. If it doesn't feel good, do it for a little while at least.

### Sun Moon Breathing

Take a shot at this to achieve the balance known as sun-and-moon breathing. To begin with, it is best if you can breathe in and out through your nose as much as possible. Breathing through the nose has three main advantages:

1. You clean the upper airway.
2. You bring the air closer to body temperature before it reaches your lungs.
3. You stimulate the brain as the air moves through the nasal cavity.

With sun moon breathing, when you breathe through the right side of your nose it's called sun breath, and when you breathe through the left side it's moon breath. Breathing this way activates both the left and right side of the brain, creating a state of balance. If you have a deviated septum or inflammation in your nose from allergies or smoking, it's likely you will notice the problem with this pose.

# Sun Moon Significance

In Hatha Yoga, the sun/moon balance is a foundational breathing technique. In fact, Hatha translates to sun/moon. Ha meaning "sun" and tha means, "moon." The "ha" or sun element has properties of being active, intense, or powerful while the "tha" or moon element has properties of being soothing, maternal, cooling.

*Moon Me, Sun Me*

Here's how to perform Sun Moon Breathing. Sit cross-legged on the floor, if you are able. Otherwise, kneel on the floor and then sit by resting the buttocks on your shins, back erect. If you like, close your eyes.

Now, start by closing off your left nostril using your left thumb. Breathe in through your right nostril. Hold that breath for a moment or two. Then exhale out through your left nostril while closing off the right nostril with a finger from your left hand.

Next, breathe back in through the left nostril, hold that breath, and then shift back to using your thumb to block the left nostril as you breathe out the through right nostril again. This completes one full cycle. Repeat two to six cycles.

Use this TOOL first thing in the morning, when you wake up, to get additional oxygen into your body. Keep some tissues handy. You might think that it's all air, but sometimes it's not.

## Many Types of yoga

There are many types of yoga. The special Targeted TOOLs above were selected to provide a few key throat-related poses for an Apnea Avenger to begin a personal healing practice. So remember, it's a practice, not a "set and forget" endeavor. Take a yoga class and add more poses. A daily yoga practice provides valuable health benefits. A practice is a living evolving program that you mature and modulate as you grow your health. It's a mindset. OSA can be overcome and can be reversed. Just put your mind to it. That's what Apnea Avengers do.

## TOOLtime

Horse wranglers "cowboy up," persons-of-interest "lawyer up," and Apnea Avengers "TOOL up" to regain and maintain their health. For us, **it's about living and not just staying alive**. Circular Breathing, the Didgeridoo, and Gum Control are targeted muscle resistance TOOLs used in or based on the findings of medical studies using targeted exercise that has been shown to lower AHI scores. Yoga offers specific poses as throat-relevant muscle resistance TOOLs that can be done standalone, combined into an existing yoga practice, or added to other routines.

Because life for most of us is busy and it's a multitasking world, some approaches work better for some than others. The point is not to prescribe what you should do, but describe, to provide ideas and options with that hope that this will make it easier for you to create a sustaining practice that you can and will do. For this is about sustaining your life, through the exercise of a sustainable practice.

# CHAPTER 11:
# Putting It All Together

## *Fifty Paces – Plus*

*Being born in Montana, I grew up camping. A few years ago, my buddies and I planned a kayaking trip around the San Juan Islands in Washington State. We were to travel light, camp on different islands each night and have a good time. By this point in my life, I knew I snored and was reminded of the fact, repeatedly, on YMCA campouts with my sons and their fifty best friends' fathers. So, to be sensible, I adopted a fifty paces rule. I always pitched my tent fifty paces from the campsite, like an outcast. During the San Juan adventure, I employed my fifty paces rule. It was working fine. Until the final night. A storm had us pinned down on an island as rain swept in on a fifty-mile-an-hour wind. We hunkered down for a day and a night. As we got close to hitting the hay, I was offered to camp right next to, or even in, the big tent. I declined, paced off my fifty paces, set up the tent and fell asleep. The next morning, I checked in with the team. Imagine my astonishment when they reported that they'd heard me all night long. Those were gale-force winds! I then had to hone my fifty paces rule: fifty-paces and downwind.*

*~W.E.H.*

# Ten Chapters In

Now that we've travelled the road of this book, you are ten chapters closer to feeling better. We've shown you the signs, the controls, and the TOOLs. It's about your body, but isn't your body a whole lot like life?

Approaching the bridge, the driver sees a sign, "Max Vehicle Weight 5,000 Pounds." Knowing that his load is over 7,000 pounds he takes a detour. He doesn't want to fall through the bridge into the canyon below. He takes action.

Hearing the hard-drive on his laptop begin to clatter and clunk, a geek plugs in a portable drive and offloads his data. Although the "brain" of his computer is failing, he's smart enough to avoid losing everything.

Humans are very smart. We make signs for each other; we notice things going wrong and take evasive action. But we aren't like trucks or computer devices. When we crash, there is no reboot. When the bottom falls out beneath us, there is a long fall into the grave. When we fail, we fail our own billions of cells. Yet that trucker is likely obese due to his sedentary life style, and he ignores the prospect of his own body crashing through the bridge that connects one day to the next. And that geek! Geesh. He is morbidly obese, too – dining perpetually on Chips and Coke, Red Bull, and Cheetos – he takes nearly zero precaution to save his own heart, though it flutters occasionally, just like his hard drive.

We are each a collection of billions of cells. But we are all also so much more than just that. We are body and mind and spirit. Our bodies have an innate desire to thrive. Our bodies depend on our minds to make good decisions in the care and consideration of what is needed to keep those billions of cells all working, coordinating, serving our purpose, our time here on earth. Some say that has to do with spirit, some not. Regardless of what you might say about that, what would your body say to your mind about the way you eat? The way you don't sleep? Does the trucker's body say, "screw the signs!" and just drive across the weak bridge, overladen? Does the geek force his hard drive to continue until it crashes and the data of his life is just... gone? What do your billions of cells have to say to you?

Sedentary lifestyles, poor life choices, ... CPU ... But you can't reboot. We wrote this book to encourage your mind, your miraculous brain, to take the decision and care for your flesh. NOW. It's up to you. Sleep or Die, remember? Lest this should begin your last chapter, it's time, with this chapter, for you to become an Apnea Avenger.

# If You Are Not Trying To Sleep

Why Try? Many Apneacs don't really understand what they are up against. For example, when the equipment breaks down, or the electricity is down, or it's just a bad night, **Apneacs may actually feel more rested in the morning if they sleep less**. Why? Well, here's a macabre fact about Apnea, something most doctors won't tell you: "If you are not trying to sleep," one Apneac shared, "then you are not gasping for air, and we all know that gasping for air is tiring. It's like drowning. I've analyzed this."

He continued with a tired look, "So by intentionally trying to sleeping less, I gasp less and am less tired than if I'd spent more hours fruitlessly, um... sleep-gasping." We advise every Apneac to treat their Apnea with CPAP. And, while we don't advise anyone to sleep less, this insight may prove helpful when your CPAP breaks down, or when you are caught without electricity or are separated from your luggage while traveling. When you are dependent upon CPAP, those things will happen. It's not if, but when.

# It's Up To You

No one can do it for you. **When the diagnosis is Apnea, the life you save will be your own. Your wife or partner can't do it for you**. Conversely, if you are the down-wind Apneac, the second-hand snorer, understand that you can only lead your snoring horse to the healing waters. (And we all know now that an Apneac snores like a horse. Or worse.)

## Threes and Sixes

What else do we know? If you've read this far, you know a lot: you know that Apnea is serious and you also know the Apnea Avenger's TOOLbox includes three drawers, or three basic approaches and TOOL sets.

- ✓ **External TOOLs drawer** – With this approach, Apnea Avengers use external TOOLs (someone or something else) that are not naturally part of the body. They are either worn, strapped on, or are modifications made to the body. External TOOLs work on either the entire system or on specific systems or parts of the body. Surgery and CPAP are examples of the TOOLs found in the External TOOLs drawer.

- ✓ **System TOOLs drawer** – With this approach, Apnea Avengers rely upon themselves to use TOOLs of knowledge and motivation to make changes to the entire bodily system. Weight Loss and Whole-Body, Global Exercise are examples of the TOOLs found in the System TOOLs drawer.

✓ **Targeted TOOLs drawer–** With this approach, Apnea Avengers rely upon TOOLs that empower them to take targeted actions, including specialized exercises, to drive specific outcomes intended to change specific parts of the body. Circular Breathing, playing a wind instrument such as the Didgeridoo, Oropharyngeal Exercises, Isometric Gum-chewing, and Throat-Targeted Yoga are all examples of the TOOLs found in the Targeted TOOLs drawer.

We will be the first to admit that there are impediments and issues with each of the TOOLs offered in this book. But to be most fair, we ask you to consider that each has their merits and challenges. We wrote this book because we observe that **the Apnea Depot looks rather cold and vacant with just a knife and a CPAP on the shelf and the droll admonition, "Lose Weight," for Apneacs that don't or won't buy**. Like corporations of billions of cells, Apneacs are people, too. We deserve options.

## No Silver Bullet

So far, there is no cure-all, no silver bullet to treat, much less heal, Obstructive Sleep Apnea (OSA) and its cruel cousins, Central Sleep Apnea (CSA) and Mixed Apnea. But we have shown you a TOOLbox filled with TOOLs, TOOLs that provide enough ammunition to take a shot at healing yourself. Practiced individually, each of these TOOLs is known to provide at least partial results. **A handful of TOOLs, like a handful of bullets, can be used in combination with the silver shotgun of determination to counter denial, and to establish your own Apnea regimen**. You'll recall from earlier chapters that there are six possible airway obstruction points between the tip of the nose and the lungs. Mathematically, this means that there are endless breath blockage combinations that can occur. For each person, this means that your **Apnea**

**plays out across your airway to form a unique blend that is a result of your physical inheritance, diet, exercise, occupation, and life style choices**. Since heavy snoring and OSA are a result of multiple factors, and since these factors may play out in one combination in one Apneac and different combinations in others, it's important to know your own Apnea-associated factors and consider each bullet for its potential to address your own specific Apnea.

## Get Smart

Be smart with your approach to overcoming OSA. What is smart? Well, the scientific method has held up pretty well over the millennium. It got humankind walking on the moon. Go with it. Measure, Try, Measure, Adjust, Compare, Do, Try, Measure, Repeat.

Remember too, that our bodies are not static. Every living thing changes over time. Your body is dynamic and will change in response to what you eat, drink, smoke and exercise. This means that you can heal yourself. It also means that, **as you age, your Apnea, and how you treat and heal it, may also need to be adjusted over time to adapt to the changing body**. Also, as you age, consider what new or additional medication are you consuming? Combinations abound. Medications may have an impact – for ill or better – on either your Apnea or your Apnea regimen.

## Step One: Get Proof Positive

The simplest first step is to ask around. Never fear! If you have a problem, someone knows something that will help. Ask the obvious questions: do you snore and do you stop breathing while sleeping? Significantly tougher is the next step: bracing for the answer. Listen and do not debate the observation. **What do you know? You were asleep!** Practice mind control. Close the mouth with your mind and listen to what those you've queried have to say. Process it, internalize it and then accept the feedback. Usually a big "thanks!" is in order. Don't shoot the messenger. Denial of untreated Apnea is a confirmed killer. Why injure your body when simple TOOLs are available?

## Not All Snorers Have OSA, Most Apneacs Snore

What's the oddest, cruelest, and bizarre twist with snoring and OSA? The snorer and Apneac are usually the very last to believe what others have observed; whether it's your nightly sleeping partner or that guy who yelled at you last weekend, who says he heard you all-night-long, from his tent three campsites away. Even in the face of mounting evidence of observed gasping for breathe, the Apneac stalls. The common response goes like this, "How can it be true when I cannot hear or see it?" It's just too hard to accept. Nowadays, with video cameras and phones everywhere at hand, proof is only one night away. If you are the down-wind Apneac or second-hand snorer, stay up and catch it on video. There are other high-tech helpers, too.

### Get More Proof

Get more proof. Depending on your situation, it may be time to get real assessments. Using technology to diagnose OSA and sleep disturbance is simpler and more effective than ever.

#### Consumer Electronics

Consumer electronics companies are making their way into the "proof" business. Now days nearly everyone has access to mobile health devices, services and applications. Within a few years there will be more. A good example of what may be possible comes from a Palo Alto startup, **Lark**. They provide a smart wristband paired with a simple **iPhone** application. The two are linked wirelessly to collect sleep data such as duration and sleep quality. The application process the data to deliver nightly sleep assessments and offers sleep coaching for better sleep hygiene. Although **Lark** detects the number of times you wake up in a night, and offers insight on OSA, it's not a medical diagnostic; but it is a first step. Two other firms, **Zeos** and **Jawbone,** offer similar consumer-grade devices for sleep observation.

*Self-Reported Surveys*

High tech monitoring too much hassle? You might prefer to try what is called a "self-reported survey," which is a fancy name for a well-designed questionnaire. Self-reported surveys are often available through wellness clinics, online, or even at work. Much like a nudge, **self-reported surveys are useful and accurate as an initial screening mechanism to deliver a "heads-up!"** Surveys hone in on your knowledge of your current health issues and then references that data to other self-reported symptoms. For example, a survey may ask questions such as "Do you have diabetes and heart disease?" or "Is your neck above size 17?" Self-reported surveys rely on patterns of Highly Correlated Afflictions to tell you more about what you already know.

# Counting Missed Sheep

How does anyone compute snoring frequency? As with a lot of other things to do with OSA, the data can be rather rustic, because it's commonly compiled as either self-reported or partner reported, sometimes recorded by device (such as a voice recorder or cell phone) or – in the case of a sleep clinic – there are advanced ways to analyze and measure snoring. Regardless where you get your data, pay attention to all the findings! Otherwise, you are likely to get fleeced... not just of your sleep, but also of your health, your life, your motivation and even your reason for being. If you have undiagnosed Apnea, or do nothing about it, you can count on your losses.

## *Home Diagnostics for OSA*

Modern home diagnostics test machines for OSA are easy to use in your home or on the road. They are sent and returned via courier. Some fit on your hand, others on your fingers, and still others on your chest or head. Order one just before Halloween and you'll have free use of a nerdy-cool costume! Some of the most modern and sophisticated units use wireless diagnostics that sense and record respiration from across the room without directly connecting to you. **With the increasing awareness of OSA and its detrimental affects on daytime wakefulness and vigilance, new companies are popping up to get these diagnostic devices quickly to the patient and get the data to you and your doctor with utmost efficiency**. So maybe you won't have to book a night with a sleep lab, or trudge to the hospital or clinic.

## *Sleep Labs*

Although home diagnostics and parallel developments in consumer electronics offer Apneacs alternatives that are as private as they are efficient, sleep labs are still an important and useful step for many others. **The advantage of a sleep lab housed in a medical site is that it will be outfitted with monitoring equipment designed to accurately detect distinguish between OSA, CSA, Mixed Apnea, or even variants such as positional OSA, and then develop a**

**response with CPAP**: and all this can often be accomplished in one night.

# Step Two: Stabilize OSA

The second step is to stabilize your breathing and sleep situation. The sooner you do this, the sooner you will begin to prevent the onslaught of over thirty OSA-related afflictions that are known to ravage the Apneac's body. **The proven, practically instantaneous path to the treatment and stabilization of Apnea is Constant Pressure (CPAP)**. CPAP machines are usually obtained through a doctor and require a prescription. Over the last twenty years, CPAP technology has matured to offer treatment and maintenance specific to each Apnea, including OSA, CSA, Mixed Apnea and rare variants.

## Hope

According to a study published online in the American Journal of Respiratory and Critical Care Medicine, researchers have found that, with early detection, followed by treatment with CPAP (continuous positive airway pressure), the brain changes caused by OSA are at least partially reversible. So if you think you or your partner may have Apnea, get help sooner than later in order to avoid or possibly reverse the worst.

### Non-Invasive First

Non-invasive approaches are the best first option for the longest lasting results. But there are other options. There are reversible, minimally invasive surgeries, like the Pillar surgery. But then,

**why not lose the weight first? THAT ALONE could DO THE TRICK**. There are extreme surgeries, such as gastric-bypass – a major internal surgery – or Mandibular Advancement, which involves sawing the jaw apart and separating the upper palate from the skull in order to reposition both the jaw and upper palate and thereby move the entire mouth forward. This extreme surgery is supposed to increase the airway and permanently eliminate Apnea, but it doesn't work all of the time. Our money is on non-invasive approaches for long lasting results.

## Already Stable?

Perhaps you have been stable for a while, maybe even twenty years. If so, it is time to get retested. Apnea is not a set-and-forget affliction: it changes with age, weight, diet, medications and neck circumference. It's up to you to make the choice to keep up with the times. Make certain that your diagnosis as well as your CPAP and your regimen reflect the real state of your Apnea.

### *Upgrade*

Upgrade your CPAP to the latest version. Get the best CPAP you can afford. Newer CPAP machines feature improved algorithms, pumps, and masks that allow breath stabilizing that is easy and safer. Stuck with a limiting deductible or full exclusion from your health plan or insurance? Shell out the money from your own pocket if need be. It could be the best thousand dollars you ever invest, especially if it saves your family the much greater expense of your early grave. Most funerals cost more that a thousand. It's your own life.

Not many forward-thinking folks have an eight-year-old computer or cell phone, but many Apneacs have CPAP machines older than that. Upgrade. Like a computer data center or even the brain, Apneacs should also have alternative backup systems in case something happens to the primary device. If you are not on a subsistence budget, get a backup machine, a battery pack, multiple masks, so you have options and are resilient. When one goes down, you can flip on the other.

Do you depend on a CPAP? Have you considered how brutal power outages lasting more than just a few hours can be? A week after the 2011 San Diego black-out, speaking before an AWAKE meeting, which is a support group for people to learn more about Apnea, stories poured forth from the group about how the two-day black out had ravaged the unprepared. Take a tip – be prepared.

# Step Three: Time to Decide if You Want to Reverse the Tide

Overcoming is defined as to "triumph over or to conquer." On the other hand, to reverse is defined as to "undo, back down, and render null and void." We say that's a fork. Don't let it stop you.

This fork in the road relates to a fundamental question: **is where I am in managing my chronic affliction, sufficient? Will it be acceptable going forward?** Stabilization is way better than its sister: untreated OSA. By stabilizing with a CPAP device, and a dental appliance, as well as options including reversible surgeries like Pillar palate-implants, your chronic condition of snoring, all the way to full-blown OSA, can subside. While using treatments like a CPAP, OSA-driven disease progression is likely arrested. Mission accomplished?

For most, the answer is yes. Either we accept the fate that befalls us from being untreated or we accept the current state of treatment, for now.

The acceptance of current treatment options might be in conjunction with a secret hope that the fabled silver bullet will come along. But for now, managing to arrest the onslaught of OSA with CPAP nighttime therapy, although that requires us to be connected to the electrical grid (or get our own solar-powered source) for the rest of our time on earth, is fine.

## ED: The BIG FAT BUMMER

As we noted earlier, iIn 2005, a team of researchers in Portugal conducted a medical study involving 98 males. The idea was to find out whether men with Erectile Dysfunction (ED) who also suffer from Apnea would experience an improvement in their ED if they were fitted with an Apnea treatment device called a CPAP. In the follow-up only one month later, over 75% of the OSA patients treated with CPAP showed remission in their ED. Hardwood had returned to the thickets of Eden.

Others don't want to take this while lying down. These are no longer Apneacs, but Apnea Avengers. It's a more aggressive stance: Like taking a shot at a dream of more independence. Now, **armed with medically studied TOOLs, Apnea Avengers want to see if they can overcome and also REVERSE OSA**. For them, their effort is worth its weight in gold.

# Step Four: Back it Down

## Avenge Yourself Against the Evil OSA

Six ways to overcome OSA offered are offered in this book, and all six require commitment, consistency and time. Of those six, five share a common denominator: they reduce neck circumference (NC). If you intend to render OSA "null and void" you must learn to develop an optimistic mindset that says, "I will do this. I can figure it out. I can take care of myself." We hope that this book will have succeeded by showing you what is possible. We look to you to provide that mind set.

Here are some final tips to propel you forward:

## Devise an Initial Approach

Devise an initial approach from the TOOLs highlighted in our book, or a combination of TOOLs found through your own research and the medical community. It's your life, so it's your plan.

## Be Consistent

Be consistent. Committing a reasonable amount of time to your diet and exercise regimen every day for a lifetime will reap health-restoring rewards versus the occasional weekend apple and stroll.

## Make it Easy

Make it easy for yourself. Do what you can. Strive, but be realistic. Most of us cannot take four hours from our day to walk, or live on a strict diet of obscure food groups.

## Self-Reliance Mindset

Adopt a self-reliance mindset. Put your future health in your hands. Take it back from the others. It's not their life. Decide now that it's yours and that you will take care of yourself. It's easy for others and even this book to "prescribe" the right exercise, diet, or even surgery. But you will live with the result. So choose. Make it YOUR own choice.

## Keep an Eye on Denial

Of course. It's just as easy for the mind to weaken and dismiss these prescriptions; the reasons are infinite. Rationalization sets in to deny any action with "I don't like that prescription." It's just another set-up, a way to give up your power over your own health. However, when you make the decision to sleep better, when you decide that you are not going to get sick or die, then you combine self-reliance with personal accountability, knowing what's really up, and that only you can make a sustainable approach to reverse your OSA. You have the information; give yourself permission to assess your best opportunities to heal, then create your own routine and try it. Continue your maintenance. Use the scientific method. Measure. Keep trying exercise, diet and healing.

## What it Takes

Do what it takes. Sleep is not a minor event in the rhythm of the body. It's critical to health. We hear people in sleep research circles talking about Sleep Hygiene; just as we teach good hygiene to children – bathe, brush your teeth, keep your clothing neat and clean, put a bandage on scrapes and scratches to prevent infection – we may now, as adults, need to educate ourselves about the importance of sleep. We need to elevate sleeping to the level of importance it deserves: Sleep or get sick, sleep or die. Or, sleep well and thrive. It's a choice.

## Imagine

Imagine what you will feel like, look like and perform like when you knock your AHI score down. Imagine knocking it down to 0. Dig out your photo album and find an older photo of you, taken when you were younger, healthier, slimmer – taken before you had Apnea. Use this photo as a marker for where you were and a level of health and fitness that you want to get back to. Post it in a place of significance. Use it as a Before and After, in reverse. Reverse Apnea, obesity, and neck circumference and go back in time, health-wise. You'll get more time in this life by being healthy.

## Measure

Measure, measure, measure. Measure your neck before and after you begin to experiment with the TOOLs. This will let you SEE when you have made progress. Measure your AHI before you begin using a TOOL, then get it measured again along the way. Yes it may be tedious, involved, because you may need a sleep diagnostic TOOL, or a sleep lab, but isn't your life worth the effort? **Set a goal to reduce your AHI by half and see what TOOLs will be your first best bet to get you there**. Measure before. Measure along the way. Make adjustments to move the needle more. Measure that. You could pretend that it's a video game, where the scoreboard is your life. Enter the game, apply the rules, strive for the goal, challenge yourself to a bigger more difficult goal, all while being highly engaged in the process. Your body will respond to the effort. Your health is the ultimate prize.

## Find YOUR Approach

Do what it takes to find an approach that works for you. Compare your symptoms, your body type, your health to the range of TOOLs offered throughout this book. If your neck size is off the charts, choose TOOLs to address that at every level. Wise choices will enhance your success.

# Observation: What is an IMpatient?

We'd like to describe the patient who looks out for his or her own health with 100% engagement, saying, "I'm the patient here." We might call this person an IMpatient. The IMpatient is a staunch self-advocate in the modern health care world. When am IMpatient receives a diagnosis, they don't simply accept their fate, they: look it up at the library, look it up on the Internet, go browse for books on the subject and don't stop by just reading a book or two. These IMpatients take control of their own healing by researching and participating in online forums, and post their questions to an audience that is worldwide; they use Linked-in, Facebook and even CrowdSource forums because they are willing to get a 2nd, 3rd, or even 4th opinion before going under the irreversible knife or submitting to a drug treatment regimen with a list of side effects which almost always includes diarrhea and death. While this stance may feel too aggressive for you, try starting with just a few questions for your doctor, such as:

✓ Can I have my results?

✓ What does this mean?

✓ What are my options?

✓ Supposing that doesn't work, is it reversible and if not, what next?

## *Nudge*

Adopt a "nudge" methodology to help. "Nudge" is a book about structuring choices into a decision architecture that improves the odds for success. Benevolent choices. For example, if Circular Breathing exercise appeals to you because you understand the critical importance of reducing your AHI, you can create the architecture to improve your success at making the better choice. Locate the Targeted TOOLs, like the didgeridoo, in a place where you will see it, and so that it's ready to be played. Or, buy a special didgeridoo just for your car, so that you can practice whenever you have extra moments away from home. A nudge is not designed to eliminate other choices, but instead to benevolently help you make the choice you know is good for you. Put things in the right place to nudge you when you get there.

## Mix and Match

Mix and match depending on your situation. If your goal is to lower your loud snoring and you are not at your "fighting weight," choose to treat the symptoms with CPAP, and then eat your way out of it with a good diet. If you are thin, weight loss is probably not your answer. Together with CPAP, your response could be Circular Breathing or Gum-Control. Use your noggin, that's what it takes.

## Keep it Simple

Don't over-complicate. Too often, complication is a self-destructive ruse that can create another reason to fall off the wagon and not get back up. Simply integrate new healthy practices into your daily life. It's as simple as putting a pull-up bar in a doorway somewhere near the middle of your home. Then you make a rule that it requires a set of ten pull-ups whenever you pass through. You might get in ten sets in a day, without even trying. Or pick up a weight ten times at that doorway. Make it easy and simple like that. Perfect practice makes perfect sense.

## Make Time

Take the time to make time for yourself. Not just Apneacs, but everyone with an excuse, will begin to tell stories about the demands of their lives; raising children, making ends meet, pleasing partners, the demands of can't-miss-TV. Hearing the excuses, you'd almost think that things were demanding you to die. Funny thing about this; **when you make yourself the priority, and stick with your plan, your momentum begins to make it happen, then all those other things are easier and you are more appreciated**. The only possible exception might be your TV: it won't care if you get sick or die.

# Reversing OSA is A Practice

Yoga, basketball, swimming, tennis, meditation or lifting weights: anyone who finds success in those activities will tell you that it "just takes practice." Reversing OSA is a practice, too. In fact, all good health is a practice. Brush you teeth. Clean your hands. Wipe. Why should stomping out an insidious affliction be any different? It is not. **It's a practice that you develop to suit your symptoms**. So, understand that the idea of a one-shot silver bullet won't work with OSA. That is your key to sleeping well and not dying as a result of No Sleep. Instead:

Practice. Hard. With determination. And there will be light at the end of the tunnel.

Can you have your cake and eat it too? The TV won't care if you get better. But it won't object when you practice your bubble-breathing therapy while watching your favorite shows. Embrace the multi-tasking world.

It's a proven fact; people can walk and chew gum at the same time. Why not walk at your "maximum fat-burning heart rate" and practice purposeful-professional-grade gum chewing? Just go light on the cake.

Make a decision to embrace TOOLs. We provide six, but there are many more possibilities. For example, buy a heart rate monitor to watch and maximize your fat-burning potential. Track your calories. Experiment. Learn what nuts do to change the mix of your fat, protein and carbohydrates. How do you feel after making a change?

Dial in on sleep with other TOOLs like **Lark** or **Zeos**. Find a TOOL that comes with sleep hygiene coaching. You may learn that you sleep too few hours for your age. What if you were to use this clue, get to bed earlier and then find that you feel better? Better is better no matter how you get there, especially if it's a non-invasive better.

## A Start Up

Geeks, take heed: think of yourself as a successful startup company. You are starting up on your own healing regimen. In the same way that successful startups iterate until they find the right track, and then continue to iterate until they crack the code of success, it is up to you to keep solving, thinking, working, exploring. The trying pays off.

## Hope Shines Bright

Since you have read this far, we've every reason to hope that you will be successful. You kept reading because you wanted to know how to heal yourself or how to help a loved-one heal. You have gained new perspectives, insights and ideas. You also know the bad news.

There is no doubt about it: Apnea is a killer of epic proportions.

Yet Apnea is recognized by too few for robbing the health and well-being from the unsuspecting.

You may have started your journey on page one innocent, unsuspecting and accepting, but now you know the deal. Your head was not designed to remain in the sand, so turn away from the banks of denial, knowing that your health situation involves treatment, and maybe even a bit of a fight. Everyone is cheering for you. Be for you, too. Fight evil back and make it shrink away. Then you become an accomplished Apnea Avenger

# A Sign In Washington, D.C.

"Due to budget cuts, the light at the end of the tunnel has been turned off."

That was posted on the wall. Make sure it isn't posted inside your head. Don't do that to yourself! Keep the light burning. OSA can be overcome.

There is hope and light at the end of the Apnea tunnel. You will feel better. Family and loved ones will applaud you, your love interest will reward you by sleeping in the same room, your billions of cells will thank you for doing your part to allow them to do their part, your brain cells will wire together, your consciousness will be raised, your life on earth will be healthy. Believe and expect this.

# It's a Mindset

It's a mindset. Be awesomely unafraid and extreme in your response to Apnea. Mount strong and stiff response to stamp out as much Apnea as you can. Perhaps you can even bop it down to zero. Be an Apnea Avenger. Make your body proud. In the beginning there was no breath, no hope, no knowledge. Now there is knowledge. There is hope. And you will have breath. Believe it. Start now.

Good night. Sleep Tight.

# afterWORD
# Apnea is No Picnic

~ Jon Warren Lentz

## Language, Apnea and Green

One of the harmonies of language is that words lend themselves to poetic depths of understanding that might not otherwise be expressible if we aren't willing to take risks. Like eating outdoors at a picnic, for example. We all know what a picnic is. It's a fun time with a blanket on the grass where we relax with food and ants. But there's another word, that sounds the same yet has a different meaning. "Pyknic" is an uncommon English word sometimes used to describe a person with a rounded build or body structure, as in, "He was very pyknic-looking: neckless and bull-bodied."

Pyknic comes from the Greek word "pykn," meaning thick. Look around; every time you see a pyknic, someone with a big neck, odds are they have Apnea. A large neck correlates with Apnea; for as we've shown in the book, Neck Circumference (NC) is the number one predictor of Apnea. These days, with an epidemic of obesity, there are a lot of folks with big necks. Apneac pyknics. It almost sounds like fun. But it isn't. Apnea is no picnic. Apnea is a killer.

In writing this book, I've taken a number of risks. And Will has indulged me. Together, we've endeavored to write an entertaining tome about a dread disease. That's because I observed in my years of teaching (and learning) that smiling people learn more and sustain their attention. Well, Apnea is no picnic, we know. So at the risk of sometimes appearing irreverent or even silly I've tried to make the work of reading a little easier with word play, pacing, and other devices one might not ordinarily find in a book about an epidemic of not breathing.

An early member of CleanTECH San Diego, when I first met Will over two years ago I was on the entrepreneurial side of that burgeoning green space, working on issues linking business and the environment. I'm still very much involved there. At that time, I knew nothing about Apnea.

Then about a year ago, Will confided about his Apnea, and that he wanted to do something about it, since he'd devoted a great deal of his last twenty years suffering from and researching about it. I think he came to me because he understood that I don't and won't participate in a-n-y-t-h-i-n-g that is not beneficial for other people. Life is just too short to simply make money.

I wanted to help, but I was concerned because meanwhile the planet is still crashing. So I agreed to do a quick book with him. We agreed to a month. Like I say, that was a year ago. There was a lot more to do than just listen, edit, and write. Already an accomplished author, I served as the mentoring co-author on this title.

"Mentoring co-author" means that, in the process of building this book based on Will's years of personal experience and guinea-pig-based research, I mentored one of the brightest minds I've known. In the process we not only remained friends but have also become better at both business and friendship.

In the course of our work together I also began to understand the linkages between personal health and the trends of civilization. Consider the breast-feeding anecdote at the start of the Diet Chapter, Chapter 8. We learned that native populations that have only recently turned away from breast-feeding are now seeing a substantial surge in Apnea as those formula babies age. This trend follows the US Apnea boom, with timing that perfectly parallels the US baby-boomer changes in breast-feeding. Here in the US, the breast fell out of favor in the very early 50's. Now the generation of the 50's is not only increasingly obese, they're often Apneacs. So it goes with subsequent bottle-fed generations. When will we learn to stop fiddling with the natural order?

The statistics on Apnea are phenomenal. It's an epidemic, a tidal wave borne on the "Tsunami of Blubber" that has overtaken our country and is slowly flooding the rest of the industrialized, wheat-and-corn-fed nations of the world.

So the other night, after an optimistic lecture by Amory Lovins, titled "Reinventing Fire," a number of environmental colleagues inquired, "Jon, why Apnea?"

I can understand the question. Like, what's Mr. Green Guy doing writing a book about everyone else's sleepless night?

Well, I'm finding that there is a poetic correlation. I lose far too much sleep wondering how we're going to put our arms around climate catastrophe. So I see the epidemic of undiagnosed Apnea as the individual analogue for eco-illogical collapse: it's parallel suffering on both the personal and planetary level, widely denied by nearly all.

Each morning, Apneacs crawl out of bed feeling like they've been hit by a truck, unaware that they've wakened all night, repeatedly, five or more times each hour, not breathing, their brains literally starved for oxygen.

So, too, with the lungs of our fevered planet! The daily loss of flora and fauna goes unnoticed. But just as every Apneac teeters towards an early death, all around the world we are choking our own species right out of existence, all day every day, and in nearly every way. We are losing species and biodiversity at a geologically unprecedented rate, while at the same time we are losing our own selves, working through a daily cloud of tedium after night after night of no sleep. At the risk of repeating myself, I say "We are practicing death as a way of life™."

We need to sleep soundly, but we also need to wake-up!

## Forward, Into Breathing Effortlessly

It's common for us to talk about life and health using the metaphor of a road. A traveler on a metaphorical road has:

- ✓ Information: maps, warning signs.
- ✓ Hazards: missing signs, bumps and dips and ditches.
- ✓ Controls: decisions and brakes and steering.

A health researcher I once knew was inclined to talk about the digestive system in terms of an automobile, comparing a regular oil change to the importance of keeping the digestive system free of pollution. But here's the problem I have with that analogy: the road is a disembodied, polluted and mechanical way of talking about the miracle that is the human body.

We are billions of cells organized to cooperate and heal and maintain us throughout the course of our lives and when we eat properly and do a modicum of exercise, we don't even have to think about it.

When the road is combined with cars to talk about health, we lose our way. Your heart, for example, is not an infernal combustion engine. Your digestive system is neither a gas tank, nor an exhaust system.

You are far more subtle and divine.

What about health and computers? These days, we hear a lot of people talking about their health in the context of the computers that have become pervasive in all aspects of our lives. Your mind is more powerful and nimble than any computer. Your heart is not a power supply. The energy that sustains your body is not electricity, but the force of life itself. To sleep is not to shutdown. And to return from a life-threatening heart attack is not at all like rebooting. To think of our bodies in terms of computers is also much, much, too disembodied!

Our bodies are the ultimate cloaks for our spirit. What we are is Flesh – Mind – Spirit. You are more than just a miracle of over a billion cells: It is a person. You.

We'd really really really like you to understand and digest that concept because you have a tremendous responsibility to own your life and to live a healthy productive one. Your co-workers, neighbors, friends, family – partners, children, parents – are all counting on you to be in this life here with them. They need you. This book is about helping you to value and care for the miracle that is you.

## Ninety Years

It's been said that some people live ninety years, but that most of those people just live one year ninety times. Over and over again. A long life. But would you call that living? An Apneac himself, one day Will said to me, "This morning, I was wondering, just how many people probably don't sleep one night, ever, and then they repeat that sleepless night, turning it over and over again every night for as many years as they live..."

Would you call a life without sleep a "good" life? Probably not! No one wants to accept any number of sleepless years under the thumb of Apnea. That's also why I chose to co-write this book.

Over the course of 20 plus years, as Will worked his way through the medical system attempting to heal his Apnea, he learned there is hope to be found even for those who have been through the wringer. And that's after several, failed, highly invasive procedures that we discuss in the book. The good news? He's become a top-notch medical researcher, probing, asking, reading and studying. But most of all, he has connected a lot of previously unconnected dots.

I believe that all of Will's suffering and all of his research has been worthwhile. Will's found the flashlights that reveal a path in the dark-night cave of Apnea. Like the combination of many small lights into a powerful beam, these lights, Will's insights, can be combined to illuminate any number of individual paths. With each light, each insight, adding a measure of control to an Apneac's plight, perhaps leading to a substantial long-term improvement, or even healing, of their Apnea. In this book, we call those insights, those lights brought to bear on the intense breathless darkness of each Apneac's cave, s. And to make our point focused and clear, we use this format: s.

## Breathing is Still Up to YOU

You, the Apneac having read this book, will have to analyze your own health situation and organize your own approach to your own healing. You have to OWN the problem. Only then can you restore your own health. So read and even re-read carefully for complete understanding. That's one purpose of this afterWORD: to send you back to page one, or to the pages you may have dog-eared or underlined, so that you will circle around and better understand the information that has taken over 20 years to bring into focus.

These TOOLs are not prescriptive. Our intention was to describe the TOOLs that may be useful, but not to prescribe their use. They are merely TOOLs that may be useful if YOU want to find a path to your own healing: ULTIMATELY, the desired results of health and healing are your own responsibility.

Of course, the danger in writing such a book is that someone is likely to fail to read, then fail to take responsibility for misreading, and consequently fail to accomplish their own healing. But the potential for healing hundreds of thousands of Apneacs far outweighs that implicit risk.

In closing, I hope you enjoyed this book. Despite or perhaps because of the topic, I've pulled out all the stops (perhaps too many) to make this the funniest, most useful and helpful book you will ever read about a dread disease affecting so many still unaware. Perhaps you can shine a light and make light of it when you talk with others who are touched by Apnea.

~J.W.L.

# ABOUT THE AUTHORS

**Will Headapohl** was raised in Montana along side the Yellowstone and the Missouri rivers with four fun sisters, one of which inherited Apnea as well. After attending Stanford, he worked in Silicon Valley for Apple, CNET, and Gateway; is a patent holder, and a co-founder of the Internet ecommerce business, BuyDirect.com. He currently resides in Rancho Santa Fe, CA where he writes, consults, rides bikes, obsesses over old and leaky Land Rovers, and plays the didgeridoo. He is married to Carlie and they enjoy raising two happy young men – Hunter and Travis. Will is an Apnea Avenger and enjoys evangelizing how to overcome Apnea.


**Jon Warren Lentz** is an autodidact polymath with a science and medical bent. A graduate of the UC Santa Cruz Classics Department, Jon's background spans the gamut of ancient and modern languages; literature and fine arts; with some business development and finance. A cross-discipline creative and serial entrepreneur, he's also an agitator. He's taught at the college level and on the national seminar circuit. He has about 6 books in print now - 3 in a dozen languages. Born and raised in the City of Orange, Jon now resides in San Diego. When not collaborating with Will, he is working to promote green businesses and sustainable solutions, through the implementation of new efficiencies from better practices to drive perpetual revenues. An early member of CleanTECH San Diego, he's a connector. He writes to elucidate unexamined truths lost beneath assumptions that are the basis of our so-called modern world.

# CITATIONS Appendix

## I: Brazilian Study Exercise Descriptions

Below are excerpts from the exercise descriptions of the Brazilian Study, "Effects of Oropharyngeal Exercises on Patients with Moderate Obstructive Sleep Apnea Syndrome," by Kátia C. Guimarães, Luciano F. Drager, Pedro R. Genta, Bianca F. Marcondes, and Geraldo Lorenzi-Filho at the Sleep Laboratory, Pulmonary Division, Heart Institute (InCor), University of São Paulo Medical School, São Paulo, Brazil.

> "Oropharyngeal exercises are derived from speech–language pathology and include soft palate, tongue, and facial muscle exercises as well as stomatognathic function exercises. The patients were instructed by one single speech pathologist (K.C.G.) to perform the following tasks:
>
> **Soft palate.** These exercises had to be repeated daily for 3 minutes and were performed once a week under supervision to ensure adequate effort. Pronounce an oral vowel intermittently (isotonic exer-cise) and continuously (isometric exercise). The palatopharyngeus, pala-toglossus, uvula, tensor veli palatini, and levator veli palatini muscles are recruited in this exercise. The isotonic exercise also recruits pharyngeus lateral wall.
>
> **Tongue.** (1) Brushing the superior and lateral surfaces of the tongue while the tongue is positioned in the floor of the mouth (five times each movement, three times a day); (2) placing the tip of the tongue against the front of the

227

palate and sliding the tongue backward (a total of 3 min throughout the day); (3) forced tongue sucking upward against the palate, pressing the entire tongue against the palate (a total of 3 min throughout the day); (4) forcing the back of the tongue against the floor of the mouth while keeping the tip of the tongue in contact with the inferior incisive teeth (a total of 3 min throughout the day).

**Facial.** The exercises of the facial musculature use facial mimicking to recruit the orbicularis oris, buccinator, major zygomaticus, minor zygoma- ticus, levator labii superioris, levator anguli oris, lateral pterygoid, and medial pterygoid muscles. The exercises include: (1) Orbicularis oris muscle pressure with mouth closed (isometric exercise). Recruited to close with pressure for 30 seconds, and right after, requested to realize the posterior exercise. (2) Suction movements contracting only the buccinator.

These exercises were performed with repetitions (isotonic) and holding position (isometric). (3) Recruitment of the buccinator muscle against the finger that is introduced in the oral cavity, pressing the buccinator muscle outward. (4) Alternated elevation of the mouth angle muscle (isometric exercise) and after, with repetitions (isotonic exercise). Patients were requested to complete 10 intermittent elevations three times. (5) Lateral jaw movements with alternating elevation of the mouth angle muscle (isometric exercise).

**Stomatognathics functions.** 1. Breathing and Speech: (1) Forced nasal inspiration and oral expiration in conjunction with phonation of open vowels, while sitting; (2) Balloon inflation with prolonged nasal inspiration and then forced blowing, repeated five times without taking the balloon out of the mouth.

2. Swallowing and Chewing: Alternate bilateral chewing and de-glutition, using the tongue in the palate, closed teeth, without perioral contraction, whenever feeding. The supervised exercise consisted of alternate bread mastication. This exercise aims for the correct position of the tongue while eating and targets the appropriate functionality and movement of the tongue and jaw. The patients were instructed to incorporate this mastication pattern whenever they were eating."

## Simplified

Inspired by this study, Will simplified these exercises to develop the following routine that, in turn, served as the basis for the "Gum Control" routine found in Chapter 10 of this book.

1. Open and close mouth slowly several times. Be sure lips are closed all the way.

2. Pucker your lips, as if for a kiss, hold, and then relax. Repeat several times.

3. Spread lips into a big smile, hold, and then relax. Repeat several times.

4. Pucker, hold, smile, hold. Repeat this alternating movement several times.

5. Open your mouth, and then try to pucker with your mouth open. Don't close your jaw. Hold. Relax. Repeat several times.

6. Close your lips tightly and press together. Relax. Repeat several times.

7. Close your lips firmly, slurp all the saliva in your mouth up onto the top of your tongue. Repeat several times.

8. Open your mouth and stick out your tongue. Be you're your tongue comes straight out of you mouth and doesn't go off to either side. Hold. Relax. Repeat several times. Work towards sticking your tongue out farther each day, while still pointing straight ahead.

9. Stick out your tongue and move it slowly from corner to corner of you lips. Hold in each corner. Relax. Repeat several times. Be sure your tongue actually touches each corner of the mouth each time.

# II: Citations by Chapter

## Chapter 1

Wikipedia. (2012, May 15). Largest Organism, 1.1. Retrieved May 16, 2012, from Wikipedia: Http>//em.wikipedia.org/wiki/Largest_organisms

Wikipedia. (2012, May 15). Positive Airway Pressure, 1.2. Retrieved May 15, 2012, from Wikipedia: http:/en.wikipedia.org/wiki/Positive_airway_pressure

Fox, S. (2011, January 1). Oropharyngeal Exam Predicts Severity of Sleep Apnea, 1.3. Retrieved May 15, 2012, from Medscape: www.medscape.com/viewarticle/751619

American College of Physicians. (n.d.). Sleep Apnea, 1.4. Retrieved from ACP Online: www.acponline.org/patients_families/diseases_conditions/sleep

## Chapter 2

Downey/III, R. (2011, December 19). Obstructive Sleep Apnea, 2.1. Retrieved May 15, 2012, from Medscape.com: www.emedicine.com/article/295807-overview

Your Lung Health. (2012, May 15). Sleep Apnea Facts, 2.2. Retrieved May 15, 2012, from YourLungHealth.com: www.yourlunghealth.org/lung_disease/sleep_apnea/facts/

Searleman. (2009, August 10). Prevalence of undiagnosed sleep apnea among surgical patients , 2.2. Retrieved May 15, 2012, from Sleep Med : www.ncbi.nlm.nih.gov/pubmed/191861

National Sleep Foundation. (2012, May 15). Number of People with Apnea in US, 2.2. Retrieved May 15, 2012, from National Sleep Foundation: www.sleepfoundation.org

Young. (1993, April 29). The occurrence of sleep disordered breathing, 2.4. Retrieved May 15, 2012, from NIH: www.ncbi.nlm.nhi.gov/pubmed/8464434

Science Daily. (2007, May 21). Sleep Apnea Increases Risk of Heart Attack or Death by 30%, 2.7. Retrieved May 15, 2012, from Science Daily: www.sciencedaily.com/releases/207/05/070520183533.htm

John J. Ratey, M. (2008). Spark: The Revolutionary New Science of Excercise and The Brain 2.5 (First Edition ed.). New York, New York, USA: Hachette Book Group.

Science Daily. (2006, November 16). Sleep Apnea Patients at Higher risk for deadly Heart Disease; Arrhythmia REM, 2.6. Retrieved May 15, 2012, from Science Daily : www.sciencedaily.com/releases/206/11/061116121443.htm

## Chapter 3

ResMed. (2012, May 15). Comorbidities, 3.1. Retrieved May 15, 2012, from ResMed: http://www.resmed.com/us/clinicians/about_sleep_and_breath ing/comorbidities/associated-risks.html?nc=clinicians

Bhangu, S. (2009, November 27). Scientists explain why breathing carbon dioxide triggers panic attack, 3.2. Retrieved May 15, 2012, from TopNews: http://www.topnews.in/scientists-explain-why-breathing-carbon-dioxide-triggers-panic-attack-2240565

Chevin. (2005, May 15). How Many Children with ADHD have Sleep Apnea. Sleep, Vol 28, No 9 , 28 (9), pp. 1041-1042.

Asthma and Allergy Foundation of America. (2012, May 15). Asthma Overview, 3.5. Retrieved May 15, 2012, from AAFA.org: http://www.aafa.org/display.cfm?id=8&cont=6

WebMD. (2012, May 15). Heat Burn and Asthma" Does GERD cause Asthma", 3.6. Retrieved May 15, 2012, from WebMD: http://www.webmd.com/asthma/guide/heartburn-asthma

National Sleep Foundation. (2012, May 15). Frequent Urination, 3.7. Retrieved May 15, 2012, from www.sleepfoundation.org/: http://www.sleepfoundation.org/article/sleep-related-problems/nocturia-and-sleep

Macey. (2008, July 1). Brain Structural Changes in Obstructive Sleep Apnea, 3.8. Retrieved 15 2012, May, from US National Library of Medicine National Institutes of Health: http://www.ncbi.nlm.nih.gov/pmc/articles/PMC2491498/

PubMed. (2008, May 5). The relationship between obstructive sleep apnea, nocturia, and daytime overactive bladder syndrome in women, 3.8. Retrieved May 15, 2012, from PubMed: www.ncbi.nlm.nih.gov/pubmed/18455544

Subramanian, S. (2009). Sleep Apnea Connected to Bruxism. 3.9 American College Of Chest Physicians, Baylor Department Of Medicine. Houston: Shyam Subramanian MD.

e! Science News. (2008, September 21). ENT/sleep apnea patients experience higher levels of depression, 3.10. Retrieved May 15, 2012, from esciencenews.com: http://esciencenews.com/articles/2008/09/21/entsleep.apnea.patients.experience.higher.levels.depression

Kumar. (2009, January 1). Neural alterations associated with anxiety symptoms in obstructive sleep apnea syndrome, 3.11. Retrieved May 2012, 2012, from US National Library of Medicine National Institutes of Health: http://www.ncbi.nlm.nih.gov/pubmed/18828142

Gonçalves. (2005, July 5). Erectile dysfunction, obstructive sleep apnea syndrome and nasal CPAP treatment, 3.12. Retrieved

2012 15, 2012, from PubMed.gov:
http://www.ncbi.nlm.nih.gov/pubmed/15946896

OZ. (2006, January 4). The Biology of Blubber, 3.13. Retrieved
May 15, 2012, from Oprah.com:
http://www.oprah.com/health/The-Biology-of-Blubber/3

Rose. (2008). Obesity Could be caused by Ear Infections or
Tonsils. American Psychological Association's 116th Annual
Convention (p. 1). 3.14 Boston: Press.

Polotsky. (2009, February 1). Obstructive Sleep Apnea, Insulin
Resistance, and Steatohepatitis in Severe Obesity. Retrieved May
15, 2012, 3.15 from American journal Of Respiratory and Critical
Care Medicine:
http://ajrccm.atsjournals.org/content/179/3/228.abstract?sid=
ee77b374-917f-468e-a58a-93964d62dbcb

Night Terrors Resource Center. (2011, January 15). 3.17 Night
Terrors and Sleep Apnea. Retrieved May 15, 2012, from Night
Terrors Resource Center:
http://www.nightterrors.org/SMF/index.php?topic=2935.0

Shives. (2011, September 27). The Many Possible Causes of
Bedwetting. 3.18 Retrieved May 15, 2012, from The Chart CNN:
http://thechart.blogs.cnn.com/2011/09/27/the-many-possible-
causes-of-bedwetting/

Harby. (2003, November 18). One Third of Sleep Apnea Patients
in Study Diagnosed With Glaucoma. Retrieved May 15, 2012,
3.20 from MedScape:
http://www.medscape.com/viewarticle/464686

Wikipedia. (2012, May 15). Periodic limb movement disorder,
3.21. Retrieved May 15, 2012, from Wikipedia:
http://en.wikipedia.org/wiki/Periodic_limb_movement_disorde
r

Luboshitzky. (2002, July 1). Decreased Pituitary-Gonadal Secretion in Men with Obstructive Sleep Apnea, 3.23. Retrieved May 15, 2012, from JCEM: http://jcem.endojournals.org/content/87/7/3394

Medtv. (2012, May 16). Sleep Disorders May Increase Risk of Developing Insulin Resistance Independent of Obesity, 3.24. Retrieved May 16, 2012, from Medtv: http://endocrine-system.emedtv.com/hypothyroidism/hypothyroidism.html

Mojon. (2002, May 12). Association between sleep apnea syndrome and nonarteritic anterior ischemic optic neuropathy, 3.24. Retrieved May 15, 2012, from PubMed: https://www.ncbi.nlm.nih.gov/pubmed/12003609

## Chapter 4

CDC. (2010, January 1). Leading Causes of Death, 4.1. Retrieved May 16, 2012, from CDC: http://www.cdc.gov/nchs/fastats/lcod.htm

Wikipedia. (2012, May 16). Sleep-Deprived Driving, 4.2. Retrieved May 16, 2012, from Wikipedia: http://en.wikipedia.org/wiki/Sleep-deprived_driving

PubMed. (2011, August 31). Diabetes, 4.3. Retrieved May 15, 2012, from PubMed Health: http://www.ncbi.nlm.nih.gov/pubmedhealth/PMH0002194/

Nainggolan. (2009, June 23). More details on arrhythmias associated with sleep apnea, 4.5. Retrieved May 16, 2012, from The Heart: http://www.theheart.org/article/981469.do

Bankhead. (2011, August 19). Nocturnal ACS Linked to Belly Fat, Disordered Sleep, 4.7. Retrieved May 16, 2012, from MedPage: http://www.medpagetoday.com/Cardiology/AcuteCoronarySyndrome/28117

NHLBI. (2010, April 8). Sleep Apnea Tied to Increased Risk of Stroke, 4.8. Retrieved May 15, 2012, from NIH: http://www.nih.gov/news/health/apr2010/nhlbi-08.htm

Young. (2000, December 20). Longitudinal study of moderate weight change and sleep-disordered breathing, 4.10. Retrieved May 15, 2012, from PubMed: http://www.ncbi.nlm.nih.gov/pubmed/11122588

## Chapter 5

Caffo. (2010, December 1). A Novel Approach to Prediction of Mild Obstructive Sleep Disordered Breathing in a Population-Based Sample: The Sleep Heart Health Study, 5.1. Retrieved May 16, 2012, from NCBI: http://www.ncbi.nlm.nih.gov/pmc/articles/PMC2982734/?tool =pubmed

Barry, D. (2012, May 16). Food Quotes, 5.5. Retrieved May 16, 2012, from FoodReference.com: http://www.foodreference.com/html/q-snickers-quotes.html

Bixler. (1998, January 1). Effects of Age on Sleep Apnea in Men, 5.8. (P. S. Department of Psychiatry, Producer) Retrieved May 16, 2012, from American Journal of Respiritory adn Critical Care: http://ajrccm.atsjournals.org/content/157/1/144.full

Mayo Clinic. (2012, May 15). Risk Factors, 5.10. Retrieved May 16, 2012, from Mayo Clinic: http://www.mayoclinic.com/health/sleep-apnea/ds00148/dsection=risk-factors

## Chapter 6

Sleeppedia. (2011, June 24). Apnea Hypopnea Index – Impact and Measurement, 6.1. Retrieved May 16, 2012, from Sleeppedia: http://sleepedia.com/apnea-hypopnea-index/

Ketcham. (2012, May 15). Epworth Sleepiness Scale, 6.5. Retrieved May 16, 2012, from Lovetoknow Sleep Disorders: http://sleep.lovetoknow.com/Epworth_Sleepiness_Scale

Wikipedia. (2012, May 15). Multiple Sleep Latency Test, 6.6. Retrieved May 16, 2012, from Wikipedia: http://en.wikipedia.org/wiki/Multiple_Sleep_Latency_Test

## Chapter 7

ResMed, Inc. (2010). 10-K 2010 Business Factors. San Diego: ResMed. 7.1

Medtronic. (2012, May 15). Pillar Procedure for Snoring and Sleep Apnea, 7.6. Retrieved May 16, 2012, from medtronic.com: http://www.medtronic.com/for-healthcare-professionals/products-therapies/ear-nose-throat/sleep-disordered-breathing-products/pillar-procedure-system-for-snoring-and-sleep-apnea/index.htm

## Chapter 8

Boyles. (2011, June 1). Weight Loss May Improve Sleep Apnea, 8.2. Retrieved May 16, 2012, from WebMD: http://www.webmd.com/sleep-disorders/sleep-apnea/news/20110601/weight-loss-may-improve-sleep-apnea

Mercola. (2010, January 10). Sugar May Be Bad, But This Sweetener is Far More Deadly, 8.4. Retrieved May 15, 2012, from Mercola.com: http://articles.mercola.com/sites/articles/archive/2010/01/02/highfructose-corn-syrup-alters-human-metabolism.aspx

Wikipedia. (2012, May 15). Nutrition, 8.5. Retrieved May 16, 2012, from Wikipedia: http://en.wikipedia.org/wiki/Nutrition

2011, November 3). Supplementation of Vitamin C and
ıcose and Improves Glycosylated Hemoglobin in Type 2
ı Mellitus: A Randomized, 8.7

ı. (2011, August 1). Does lack of sleep cause diabetes?, 8.8.
ıved May 16, 2012, from Cleveland Clinc Journal of
ıcine: http://www.ccjm.org/content/78/8/549.full

ıble-Blind Study, 8.7. Retrieved May 16, 2012, from Hindawi:
ıp://www.hindawi.com/journals/aps/2011/195271/

Vard. (2012, May 15). Fat Facts: Good Fats vs. Bad Fats, 8.9.
Retrieved May 16, 2012, from WebMD:
http://www.webmd.com/food-recipes/features/good-fats-bad-fats

## Chapter 9

Grontved. (2011, June 15). Television viewing and risk of type 2
diabetes, cardiovascular disease, and all-cause mortality: a meta-analysis., 9.1. Retrieved May 16, 2012, from JAMA:
http://www.ncbi.nlm.nih.gov/pubmed/21673296

John J. Ratey, M. (2008). Spark: The Revolutionary New Science
of Excercise and The Brain 2.5/9.2 (First Edition ed.). New York,
New York, USA: Hachette Book Group.

Sports Fitness Advisor. (2012, May 15). Determine Lactate /
Anaerobic Threshold, 9.6. Retrieved May 16, 2012, from Sports
Fitness Advisor: http://www.sport-fitness-advisor.com/anaerobicthreshold.html

Zabell. (2011, June 15). Is Cyling Better Than Walking, 9.7.
Retrieved May 16, 2012, from LiveStrong.com:
http://www.livestrong.com/article/210806-is-cycling-better-than-walking-to-lose-weight/

Johansson. (2011, June 1). Longer term effects of very low energy diet on obstructive sleep apnoea, 9.10. Retrieved May 16, 2012, from BMJ: http://www.bmj.com/content/342/bmj.d3017.full

## Chapter 10

Wikipedia. (2012, May 15). Circular Breathing, 10.1 Retrieved May 16, 2012, from Wikipedia: http://en.wikipedia.org/wiki/Circular_breathing

Wagner. (2009, June 02). High resistance wind instrument may reduce OSA, 10.2 Retrieved May 15, 2012, from AASM: www.aasmey.org/articles.aspx?id=1312

Svanborg. (2011 November 22). Long-term snoring can cause nerve damage in throat, 10.3. Retrieved May 16, 2012, from Linkopings University: http://www.liu.se/?l=en

Guimaraes. (2009, May, 15).10.4 Effects of Oropharyngeal Excercises on Patients with Moderate OSA. Retrieved May 16, 2012, from NIH: http://www.ncbi.nlm.nih.gov/pubmed/19234106

## Chapter 11

Lark Technologies. (2012, MAY 15). LARK MAIN, 11.1. Retrieved MAY 15, 2012, from LARK: www.lark.com

Made in the USA
Lexington, KY
18 October 2012